# THE
# CIRCADIAN
# DIABETES
# CODE

# ALSO BY SATCHIN PANDA, PHD

*The Circadian Code*

# THE CIRCADIAN DIABETES CODE

Discover the Right Time to
Eat, Sleep, and Exercise to Prevent and
Reverse Prediabetes and Diabetes

## Satchin Panda, PhD

RODALE

NEW YORK

Published in the United States by Rodale Books, an imprint of Random House, a division of Penguin Random House LLC, New York.
rodalebooks.com

RODALE and the Plant colophon are registered trademarks of Penguin Random House LLC.

Library of Congress Cataloging-in-Publication Data
Names: Panda, Satchin, author.
Title: The circadian diabetes code : discover the right time to eat, sleep, and exercise to prevent and reverse prediabetes and diabetes / Satchin Panda, PhD.
Description: New York : Rodale, 2021. | Includes bibliographical references and index.
Identifiers: LCCN 2021021535 (print) | LCCN 2021021536 (ebook) |
ISBN 9780593231876 (hardcover) | ISBN 9780593231883 (ebook)
Subjects: LCSH: Diabetes—Prevention. | Non-insulin-dependent diabetes. |
Circadian rhythms—Health aspects.
Classification: LCC RC660.4 .P36 2021 (print) | LCC RC660.4 (ebook) |
DDC 616.4/62—dc23
LC record available at https://lccn.loc.gov/2021021535
LC ebook record available at https://lccn.loc.gov/2021021536

ISBN 978-0-593-23187-6
Ebook ISBN 978-0-593-23188-3

Printed in the United States of America

Jacket design by Pete Garceau

10 9 8 7 6 5 4 3 2 1

First Edition

To my mother, Geetanjali

# Contents

# ACKNOWLEDGMENTS

In 2015, when we published our first human study showing that the average person eats for 15 hours or longer each day, and that reducing this eating interval to 10 hours can promote weight loss, improve sleep, and increase the sense of energy, I received a pleasant surprise. Dr. Eric Topol of the neighboring Scripps Research Translational Institute tweeted our study findings. Dr. Topol is a world-renowned cardiologist who immediately saw the potential of our research on time-restricted eating, which is now more commonly known as intermittent fasting, or IF.

We assumed right away that what was good for weight loss would be highly effective in reducing the risk for diabetes and heart disease. It seems the public was on the same page. Soon thereafter, I fielded calls from patients and physicians asking for advice on how to implement IF for weight loss and diabetes management. But we needed more data from clinical studies overseen by physicians. Within weeks, Dr. Julie Wei-Shatzel started prescribing a 10-hour IF for her patients with diabetes or prediabetes along with the typical medications. After a few months, she informed me that her patients were making progress in managing their blood glucose and in many cases reducing their medications. Those early results from a physician encouraged me to start collaborating with researchers working in different universities around the world to test the impact of IF on people at high risk for developing diabetes, people with prediabetes, or those with diabetes.

About a year later, in 2016, I was lucky enough to have Dr. Emily Manoogian, a postdoc trainee, join my lab. She already had a PhD in circadian rhythm research and was eager to lead clinical human research in my group. I am immensely thankful for my collaborators who showed early curiosity about IF and took a big risk in trying out a new idea to manage diabetes. They include Dr. Pam Taub, Dr. Tinh-Hai Collet, Dr.

Lisa Chow, Dr. Leonie Heilbronn, Dr. Krista Varady, and Dr. Blandine Laferrère. Several scientists, including Dr. Courtney Peterson, Dr. Kristine Færch, Dr. Josiane Broussard, and Dr. John Hawley, also consulted with me to start their independent research into IF and diabetes. In parallel, several laboratories around the world started assessing the impact of IF on aspects of diabetes risk or its complications. I am immensely thankful for these early testers of IF.

Our pilot study on the impact of a 10-hour IF on metabolic syndrome started in collaboration with Dr. Pam Taub at the University of California, San Diego. In 2018, after our first metabolic syndrome patient completed his 12-week IF program, Dr. Taub was ecstatic about the results. The patient had reduced his blood sugar and blood pressure to normal levels and had lost enough weight from his belly to have reduced his waist circumference by 2 inches. I was happy, but I was puzzled. Dr. Taub is a famous preventive cardiologist, and she treats dozens of patients with metabolic syndrome every week. Many of her heart patients are also diabetic. I thought doctors like her were curing people with drugs, but she told me that her typical patients were not seeing much benefit from their medications, or when they did see some benefits, they also complained about adverse side effects. But the patient who did IF saw multiple benefits and had no complaints. In fact, he promised to continue his IF as a new lifestyle. The same story was repeated again and again with Dr. Taub's study and in the studies of other collaborators. This is when I knew that we had come across something special.

The decision to write this book came quite abruptly. In 2018, I received a Pioneer funding award from the Robert Wood Johnson Foundation (RWJF) to advance the knowledge of circadian rhythms and IF among clinicians and basic scientists by facilitating their research through the myCircadianClock app. I was attending a workshop related to science communication to nurture a culture of health at the RWJF campus in Princeton, New Jersey. By the end of the conference, I was jazzed up about communicating our latest findings. And that is when my friend Pam Liflander drove down from Connecticut to have a chat over dinner. We could not have the dinner meeting at a more opportune time. She convinced me that I should write this book and she would help me, just as she had done so well with my first book, *The Circadian Code*.

The outline for the book took shape during many dinner-table discussions with my family. My wife, Smita, and daughter, Sneha, would listen patiently to my scientific explanation and nudge me toward a simple clarification. Every once in a while, when my curious mother would visit me, she would also join the discussion by sharing her own journey with IF to reverse her diabetes. My family's patience with my long hours in the lab and frequent travels, and their constant support, has been priceless.

My editor, Donna Loffredo, and her team at Penguin Random House have been a pleasure to work with. My agent, Carol Mann, played an integral role in getting the project off the ground.

I am thankful to the Salk Institute for Biological Studies, where scientific excellence, symbiosis, and a strong drive to make foundational breakthroughs that can leave a lasting impact on the planet have been fueling my research. The work of the founder, Dr. Jonas Salk, is specifically inspiring for me: his development of the polio vaccine proves the powerful message that prevention is the best cure. The Salk Institute has given me unwavering support to do many unconventional experiments. My principal collaborators and scientific colleagues at Salk include Dr. Ron Evans and Dr. Marc Montminy, who introduced me to the molecular connections between circadian rhythms and nutrition metabolism, which form the foundation for understanding how nurturing your circadian rhythm is central to diabetes prevention and management. Dr. Reuben Shaw, Dr. Alan Saghatelian, and Dr. Joe Ecker have helped me with my circadian rhythm research in understanding how gene activities at different times of the day influence metabolism.

Outside of Salk, my collaborations and discussions with leaders in the area of intermittent fasting, circadian rhythm, metabolism, and diabetes include Dr. Dan Drucker, Dr. Mark Mattson, Dr. Johan Auwerx, Dr. Valter Longo, Dr. Eric Verdin, and Dr. Joe Takahashi, all of whom xiiACKNOWLEDGMENTS

helped integrate the science behind Time-Restricted Eating (TRE) and circadian rhythm with the science of diabetes.

I am truly fortunate to work with a great group of students and trainees. Their hard work and long hours in the lab to break their own circadian code made it possible to test many of the ideas described in this book. I am especially thankful to Hiep Le, Dr. Christopher Vollmers, Dr. Megumi Hatori, Dr. Shubhroz Gill, Dr. Amandine Chaix, Dr. Amir Zarrinpar, Dr. Ludovic Mure, Dr. Luciano DiTacchio, Terry Lin, and Dr. Shaunak Deota.

I am also grateful for research funding from the National Institutes of Health, U.S. Department of Defense, Department of Homeland Security, Leona M. and Harry B. Helmsley Charitable Trust, Robert Wood Johnson Foundation, Pew Charitable Trusts, American Federation for Aging Research, Paul F. Glenn Center for Biology of Aging Research, American Diabetes Association, American Heart Association, World Cancer Research Fund International, Joe W. and Dorothy Dorsett Brown Foundation, William H. Donner Foundation, Auen Foundation, Chapman Foundation, Joe and Clara Tsai Foundation, Irwin and Joan Jacobs, Dan Tierney, and Barbara Friedman.

Finally, through the myCircadianClock.org website and research app, thousands of people have come to learn about their own circadian rhythms and have shared their positive health changes achieved by following the lessons presented in this book. I am grateful to all of them.

# INTRODUCTION

If you or a loved one has recently been diagnosed with prediabetes or diabetes, you are not alone. According to the U.S. Centers for Disease Control and Prevention (CDC), one in ten Americans has diabetes, and one in three is likely to have prediabetes right now. Just by reading this book, you are taking a very important step forward in managing your health.

Having a doctor tell you that you have prediabetes, or Type 2 diabetes is almost like running a temperature greater than 100.4°F. It's a sign that some aspect of your health is off balance, and if you don't pay attention, it can become much worse, potentially leading to life-threatening complications. Not only is diabetes linked to other chronic health conditions like obesity, heart disease, and Alzheimer's disease, but it is also one of the most devastating underlying conditions related to intensifying infectious diseases such as COVID-19.

Yet we know that even with diabetes, some days we feel better than other days. When we stop to think about it, those better days are typically the ones when we have slept well, ate nutritious foods, and even exercised. In the very same way, with these very same tools, anyone can learn how to control their diabetes, and possibly even reverse a diagnosis.

I'm on the forefront of circadian rhythm research, which is the science of our biological clocks. In my first book, *The Circadian Code*, I showed readers all over the world how every cell in the human body has a clock and keeps a schedule of when it is the optimal time for it to function. My research has fueled a whole new way of eating, which I call *time-restricted eating* (TRE), and is more commonly known as *intermittent fasting* (IF). Basically, my research shows that when it comes to weight loss, it's not only what you eat that makes a difference. To lose weight, it's equally important to make good decisions about *when* you eat. My protocol not only works for weight loss; it also optimizes every cell in the body, including those that monitor blood glucose. If we nurture our circadian rhythm, it in turn nurtures our health. If you can control when you eat, you can reverse your prediabetes, manage your long-term or recently diagnosed Type 2 diabetes, and lose weight along the way. By doing so, you can also enhance every other aspect of your health.

How do I know all this? Just ask my mother.

## MEET MRS. PANDA

I am lucky enough not to have prediabetes or diabetes—yet. However, I know that I have a high risk for developing diabetes and heart disease just by being from South Asia. For the past eight years, I have adopted an intermittent fasting lifestyle in which I try to eat within a fixed 10-hour window most days. This has helped me shed some extra weight. But the best results from intermittent fasting have been with my mother.

Seven years ago, my mother noticed the blood sugar numbers on her annual physical exams were creeping up. Over the next two years, her exams showed that her blood sugar was continuing to rise; in other words, she was approaching a diabetic state. Even though her doctor wasn't really worried, she panicked because she knows the damage diabetes can cause. She had seen too many friends and relatives who ignored the early signs of the disease, and even after taking daily medications for years, they slowly developed heart disease, kidney disease, blindness, and even dementia. My mother was also less than thrilled about the idea of living with diabetes, having to carefully monitor what she ate at every single meal.

When she first told me the news, we talked about her daily diet and exercise routine, because it is well known that the foods you eat and the amount you exercise can influence your blood sugar levels. Yet even though she was already doing everything right, the results weren't adding up. As a vegetarian, she would eat more than the recommended portions of fruits and vegetables every day, and she would take a daily walk in the evenings. She was also fasting at least once a week for religious reasons, while on other days she ate dinner by 8:00 p.m. But I noticed occasionally, at least two or three times a week, she would have a cup of tea with sugar and milk around 9:00 p.m. if she visited any of our relatives; it was difficult for her to decline a late-night snack.

I knew from my previous research that by eliminating this occasional and seemingly benign late-night snacking, she may be able to see some improvements in her blood glucose. When I first told her this, she laughed at me. Besides, her doctor and other health professionals could not be convinced that these small late-night meals were the culprit, pushing her toward diabetes.

A few months later I convinced her to visit me in the United States. When she lived with me for the next several months, she adopted my stricter rule of no food after 6:00 p.m. In the morning, she ate her breakfast around 9:00 a.m. That pattern created a daily eating window of 9 hours. Over the next several weeks, she told me that she had never felt better. And when she returned to India and continued eating this way, her blood sugar levels declined to below a prediabetic level. After five months, her fasting blood glucose was hovering near a healthy range. Best of all, for the past five years, she's been able to stay healthy and off all medications—just by keeping to the protocol.

Since then, I have repeated this experiment in more than a dozen clinical trials. My group has worked not only with patients who have prediabetes but also those suffering from high cholesterol and high blood pressure. We always find that those who can follow a 10-hour IF can substantially improve their health.

## LET YOUR CLOCK CONTROL YOUR BLOOD SUGAR

Now it's time to try this experiment together. You can be in complete control of your blood sugar by living in alignment with your circadian rhythm. Not only is it easy, but also every aspect of your health will get better. In this book, you'll learn when to eat, when to exercise, when to sleep, when to work, and when to take your medications, if necessary. If this program sounds simple, that's because it is.

Your doctor may tell you to eat less, exercise more, and stay away from sugar and carbohydrates. There is sufficient research to substantiate these recommendations. However, the problem is in the compliance. Experts know that to follow these recommendations, you have to count calories for every meal you eat, track and avoid the foods that are known to raise your blood sugar, and count how many miles you walk or run. If you can do this, great; many people with prediabetes or diabetes begin this type of program and see some benefits within a month or two. But more often than not, the regimen becomes too difficult to sustain for a long time. Even though these are good habits to form, they are too arduous. This is where my research on circadian rhythm and time-restricted eating is opening new avenues for treating diabetes.

Research on circadian rhythm has shown that blood glucose regulation is more complex than we had known before. When we eat, when we exercise, and how much or when we sleep have a big impact on our blood glucose. By following this program, you may achieve your goals without counting a single calorie.

In addition, you'll learn that IF has numerous other benefits on various organ systems, immune systems, and the brain, including weight loss. When it is practiced over a few months, you can retrain your liver and fat tissues to break down unwanted fat and cholesterol. In preclinical studies, we have found a clear sign of a reduction in risk for heart disease. These findings are very important, because someone with diabetes has the same risk for heart disease or heart attack as a nondiabetic person who has already had one heart attack. We also have found that IF improves kidney function. One common diabetes complication is chronic kidney disease and kidney failure. And by losing weight and enhancing immunity, you are doing the two best things possible for avoiding COVID-19 complications.

## HOW THIS BOOK WORKS

During the last few years, as IF became popular in the mainstream media, many people who had heard me on a podcast, followed me on Twitter, or read *The Circadian Code* would try IF and contact me with their success stories or to seek advice on how to implement IF in their own life. As I am not a physician, I would always advise them to consult with their doctors regarding my suggestions. Slowly I realized that my physician colleagues are busy writing prescriptions, and even if they wanted to help their patients establish an optimum lifestyle to manage disease, either they didn't have enough time or weren't familiar with the nascent science of circadian rhythm. But it also became apparent that every patient needs a lot of guidance and information between their visits to doctors' offices on how to live a healthy life. That is why I decided to write this book.

This book serves three purposes. It is a source of essential knowledge about the new science of circadian rhythm and how it relates to controlling blood sugar. It provides an integrated practice for both IF and optimizing your entire circadian rhythm within your lifestyle. And it shares the experiences of all different kinds of people who practice IF and relates how they tackled the challenges to ultimately improve their diabetes. The beauty of circadian rhythm and IF is that anyone, irrespective of age, sex, ethnicity, or income level, can implement it in their own life. I hope you will share this knowledge with your family and community so that we can create and sustain a culture of (circadian) health.

In Part I, you will learn about both the basics of circadian science and the latest research regarding diabetes and what I call "the sinister friends of diabetes," heart disease and obesity. You will be able to assess your current risk for developing diabetes, and what you need to focus on if your doctor has already given you this diagnosis. You will also see how living out of alignment with your natural circadian rhythm may be negatively impacting your risk factors or the way you are managing your diabetes right now.

In Part II, you will learn how to get back into better alignment. You will discover how to be successful with IF, which is a critical tool for better regulating your blood sugar levels. You will not only determine when is the best time to eat but also what you should be eating. As you probably know, exercise and good sleep are also critical. Now you will learn when is the best time to exercise and which types of exercise are best for managing diabetes. Lastly, you will learn more about the importance of sleep and how to limit light exposure at night: each play an important role in managing diabetes.

In Part III, you will first learn how to understand exactly what your doctor is trying to tell you during your annual checkups. You will then learn how to make the most of every appointment with your doctor and how to introduce him or her to circadian science so you can better manage your diabetes. Then, you will put everything you've learned to the test, and participate in a 12-week health challenge that will get you the results you are looking for. It is hoped you'll believe as I do that living in alignment with your circadian rhythms is the easiest way to maintain good health over the long run.

What do you have to lose? Let's get started.

**PART 1**

# Understanding Diabetes
# and the Circadian Code

## CHAPTER 1

# Diabetes Explained

The diabetes discussion begins and ends with food. Our meals contain one or more of three *macronutrients:* carbohydrates, proteins, and fats. As soon as we eat, the digestive juices in our gut break these macronutrients into the smallest molecules so that our cells, all over our body, can use them. Fats are broken down to simpler fatty-acid molecules; proteins are broken down to amino acids; and carbohydrates are ultimately broken down to sugars such as glucose. These fatty acids, amino acids, and glucose molecules are released into the bloodstream, where they travel to the different organs to power our cells, repair them, and make new cells.

For most of us, carbohydrates are at the heart of each of our meals: cereal for breakfast, a sandwich for lunch, pasta or rice with dinner. So, it is not surprising that out of the three key macronutrients, we have an abundance of sugar/glucose molecules floating in our bloodstream. Sometimes, our meals are so ladened with sugar that we couldn't possibly use all the sugar that we eat immediately. So, just like we store gas in our car's gas tank, the body has created a way to store glucose and the other macronutrients we eat and use them judiciously between meals. For instance, a can of juice or soda typically has 39 grams of sugar, and if all of it entered our blood without getting absorbed in our cells and organs, our blood sugar would rise to a life-threatening level. Therefore, within minutes of eating, hormones sense the arrival of carbohydrates and prepare the liver, muscles, and fat tissues to store most of the carbohydrates or sugar we just ate. The sugar is stored in the form of glycogen and, to some extent, body fat. Fatty acids are stored as fat, and amino acids are stored as proteins.

Almost every cell in our body and brain loves glucose as a source of energy. In fact, our body constantly needs energy—much more often than the number of times a day we eat. So, just as we have a process for storing nutrients, our body has different mechanisms to sense our level of physical and mental activity, and releases just enough stored energy to support it. Between meals, our body has to predict our energy demand and accurately release just the right amount of glucose from the stored glycogen. When the glycogen store goes low, the body can then break down stored fat to supply energy to many cells. Our body can also use some stored proteins and convert them to glucose.

These two mechanisms—how we both store and release glucose—are at the heart of controlling how much sugar is in our bloodstream at any given time. When we can maintain this delicate balance, we have health. But when blood glucose levels are too high after a meal, or the body releases too much glucose from storage on demand, we have problems.

## ONLY 5 GRAMS OF SUGAR

A healthy adult body is designed to have between 4 and 6 grams of sugar in the blood—just one teaspoon—no matter if you have just finished a heavy meal, are in the middle of a marathon run, are deep asleep, or have not eaten for a day. Just like a fish in a fish tank, where even the slightest change in water quality can make the fish sick, every cell in our body performs best within a narrow range of blood sugar. When the exquisite mechanisms that sense and regulate our blood glucose levels go even slightly off, there is a grave danger that brain and body cannot perform well. If your blood sugar falls below 3.5 grams, you may notice that your vision begins to blur, or you feel dizzy. This is referred to as *hypoglycemia*.

Since we almost always eat more carbohydrates/sugars than we need to support a healthy blood sugar level, and our body has plenty of stored carbohydrates (glycogen) and alternate sources of glucose (protein), most problems with blood glucose regulation result in too much sugar in our blood. If your blood sugar rises above 6 grams and stays there for long periods of time, you will develop diabetes.

But let's not get ahead of ourselves. First, let's talk about what happens to your health when things go right. When your body is working optimally, it can regulate blood glucose levels precisely through a variety of players that mostly fall into four major groups: energy sensors, hormones, hormone sensors, and gates that allow glucose to pass through the cells. The most important of these are the hormones and their sensors. And the most important hormone is *insulin,* which is produced from a few thousand cells in our pancreas. Insulin's "hormone sensor," or *receptor,* is present in almost every cell in our body.

When we eat, digested carbohydrates from our food rush into the blood and our blood glucose level quickly goes up—within minutes. This blood glucose increase is sensed by the pancreas, which releases insulin. Insulin is responsible for opening the door on every cell to let in the glucose so it can be used for energy. It's like the electronic signal from your garage door opener that connects to a receiver (the insulin receptor) to open the garage door so you can drive your car (glucose) into the garage (a cell). The same insulin code can open nearly all the doors in all the cells, including the liver, muscle, and fat cells. This is important because these cells absorb and store most of our excess carbs so that your blood glucose level comes back to normal within an hour or two after a meal.

You may need to release some glucose from storage to power your body and brain. Usually this happens several hours after a meal, when the easiest available glucose begins to decline, or if your body suddenly needs extra energy, such as when you are running or doing strenuous work. Our brain alone consumes up to 5 grams of glucose every hour. If an average-size adult is briskly walking (4 miles/hour), they are using an energy equivalent of 1 gram of glucose every minute. These conditions require releasing some glucose from the stores, or if the store is running low, making glucose by breaking down protein. Just like insulin signals the glucose to enter cells for storage, a separate set of hormones that sense hunger or stress signal the storage tank to release just enough glucose to meet the energy need without letting the blood glucose level rise too high.

Now let's look at what happens in the hours between meals. After you've eaten there is a changing of the guard—the hunger hormones shut down so that the flow of glucose from the liver is stopped. You will be accessing the glucose from the food you just ate. The eating hormone, which is insulin, turns on so that the rising blood glucose from the meal you ate is now sent to the liver, muscle, and fat to avoid blood glucose rising too high. The cycle continues every time you eat.

---

**YOU ARE NOT ALONE**

Almost one in three adults in the United States and almost one in four adults around the world have either diabetes, elevated blood glucose, or are at risk of developing elevated blood glucose.[1] That means you are not alone. It is very likely that someone you know (your parents, siblings, children, or a close friend) has this problem. So, when you master the techniques to bring your health under control, you can also help your loved ones reach their full physical, mental, and emotional potential.

---

## THERE ARE DIFFERENT TYPES OF DIABETES

When blood sugar cannot be controlled, we develop one of several forms of diabetes. It is important to know which type of diabetes you have been diagnosed with so that you can accurately monitor it and treat it more effectively. Your body may not be producing enough insulin, or your insulin sensors/receptors may have gone defective. Or, there may be certain conditions in which an imbalance of other hormones may affect your body's ability to regulate glucose. Based on these causes, there are at least five different types of diabetes known today. All of the suggestions in this book may apply to you, regardless of what form of diabetes you are dealing with. The only difference is the way your health improves.

TYPE 1 DIABETES. In most instances, Type 1 diabetes develops early in childhood, but for some people it can happen later in life. The cause of Type 1 diabetes is believed to have nothing to do with diet or lifestyle. Instead, it is a true autoimmune disease resulting in insulin deficiency. The immune system gets confused and thinks the insulin-producing cells in the pancreas are foreign invaders. The body starts attacking and destroying these precious cells, and the result is that the pancreas never produces enough insulin to move glucose into the cells where it is needed. Symptoms of Type 1 diabetes include frequent urination, slow-healing cuts and bruises, extreme thirst, dry mouth, fatigue, weakness, and increased appetite combined with weight loss.

TYPE 2 DIABETES. This form can develop at any age, although it is most prevalent in adulthood. It occurs when the body doesn't use insulin properly, and the pancreas makes extra insulin to compensate, but is unable to keep up with the demand. Symptoms of Type 2 diabetes include frequent urination, extreme thirst and hunger, slow-healing cuts and bruises, drowsiness, low energy, pain or numbness in the arms and legs, vision changes, sweet-smelling breath, and unexplained nausea or vomiting.

GESTATIONAL DIABETES. Usually, this is a temporary form of diabetes that occurs during the second or third trimester of pregnancy. The body does not produce adequate amounts of insulin. Its symptoms include extreme thirst, frequent urination, fatigue, nausea, vaginal and bladder infections, vision changes, and slow-healing cuts and bruises.

DIABETES DUE TO OTHER CAUSES. Some forms of diabetes are specifically related to other health issues. These conditions can include diseases of the pancreas, such as cystic fibrosis or pancreatitis, and drug/chemical-induced diabetes, which can occur if someone is taking glucocorticoids, is being treated for HIV/AIDS, or has had an organ transplant. It occurs because the pancreas stops producing normal amounts of insulin, causing insulin deficiency and the same symptoms as Type 1 diabetes.

PREDIABETES. According to the Centers for Disease Control and Prevention (CDC), close to 88 million American adults—more than one in three—have prediabetes.[2] Of those with prediabetes, 90 percent don't know they have the condition because there are no serious symptoms. It occurs when blood glucose levels are higher than normal (>100 mg/dL), but not high enough to be classified as full-blown diabetes (<126 mg/dL). If left untreated, prediabetes can progress to Type 2 diabetes. However, if treated, it can completely resolve itself. If you've received this diagnosis, you are in the best position to improve your health and completely reverse prediabetes by using this program and making healthy changes to the way you live right now. These steps include managing your weight, exercising at the right time of day, eating healthier, quitting smoking and, most important, aligning your eating/sleeping cycle to your innate circadian code.

Be sure to ask your doctor what your exact blood sugar test results are when he or she tells you that you have prediabetes; that way, you can track your progress in reversing the trend and attaining better health.

## RISK FACTORS TO CONSIDER

Diabetes doesn't come out of nowhere. Take age, which is a significant risk factor. As we get older, every part of our body ages, including the pancreas; an old pancreas may not produce enough insulin. Or, the cells become insensitive to insulin, so they do not respond correctly as we get older. We also know that men have a higher incidence of diabetes than women; it's thought that the female sex hormones protect against diabetes to some extent. Having certain genes, and specific combinations of genes, can also predispose someone to diabetes, which is why people of certain ethnicities are at a higher risk for diabetes, independent of one's habits. This means that Asian Americans, Pacific Islanders, African Americans, Latinos, and Native Americans are genetically predisposed to diabetes, regardless of their typical diet or lifestyle.

Diabetes treatments are personalized to match a person's overall health and what side effects they are likely to experience from diabetes medications. This means that depending on your health, age, sex, weight, and race, you may be treated very differently from someone else in your family. Let's use percentages as a method for comparison. For example, a parent or grandparent in their 70s or 80s who has been living with diabetes for the past 20 years, and who has other health conditions, may be put on a treatment regimen to maintain the blood glucose levels at around 8%, because the medications to lower the blood glucose to 7% or 6% may do more harm, owing to adverse side effects. For someone in their 50s diagnosed with Type 2 diabetes and not having other health complications; the doctor may set a treatment target to bring their blood glucose down to 7%.

Now, if you are diagnosed with a blood glucose level of 6.5%, your older friends may tell you that 6.5% is nothing compared to what they have been struggling with. And if you are diagnosed with prediabetes with a blood glucose of 5.8%, someone else may even tell you to completely ignore your blood report. However, you can't compare your results to those of your relatives. If you ignore your prediabetes or early-stage diabetes, thinking you are not "that bad yet," and you do not make any attempt to change your lifestyle or get on medication, you will end up at a stage of diabetes where you can no longer simply "get back to normal."

## HOW MUCH DO YOU WEIGH?

Not everyone who is overweight will develop diabetes. And not everyone with diabetes is overweight. However, weight is an important risk factor that is within our control. As we gain weight, the pancreas doesn't proportionately increase in size, making it less effective at producing enough insulin to support the entire body. What's more, the extra fat cells we acquire with weight gain interfere with insulin function. These two reasons are why weight gain poses an increased risk for diabetes.

The following chart shows the average height-to-weight ratio that signals an increased risk for developing diabetes.

| Height | Your Risk for Diabetes Increases If You Weigh More Than |
|---|---|
| 4′10″ | 119 lbs. |
| 4′11″ | 124 lbs. |
| 5′ | 128 lbs. |
| 5′1″ | 132 lbs. |
| 5′2″ | 136 lbs. |
| 5′3″ | 141 lbs. |
| 5′4″ | 145 lbs. |
| 5′5″ | 150 lbs. |
| 5′6″ | 155 lbs. |
| 5′7″ | 159 lbs. |
| 5′8″ | 164 lbs. |
| 5′9″ | 169 lbs. |
| 5′10″ | 174 lbs. |
| 5′11″ | 179 lbs. |
| 6′ | 184 lbs. |
| 6′1″ | 189 lbs. |
| 6′2″ | 194 lbs. |
| 6′3″ | 200 lbs. |
| 6′4″ | 205 lbs. |

## SHOULD I GET TESTED FOR DIABETES OR PREDIABETES?

We know that the way we live our lives either increases the risk for diabetes or discourages it. These are the factors we can—and should—control. Many of the following lifestyle habits—like physical activity, how much sleep you get each night, when you eat your last meal of the day, and if you do shift work—factor into your risk load. This is why some people who are thin and otherwise healthy are shocked to discover they have been diagnosed with diabetes. But really, there is always an underlying cause.

Give yourself one point for any of the following that applies to you. You should be screened if you have five or more of the following diabetes risk factors:

- Are Asian American, Pacific Islander, African American, Latino, Native American

- Are a man

- Are a woman with polycystic ovary syndrome (PCOS)

- Are overweight (see chart, opposite)

- Have a family history of diabetes

- Have a history of cardiovascular disease

- Have an HDL cholesterol level (the "good" cholesterol) of 35 mg/dL or lower and/or triglyceride level of 250 mg/dL or higher

- Have had gestational diabetes or have given birth to a child weighing more than 9 pounds

- Are an overnight shift worker or live a lifestyle where you stay awake for 2 to 3 hours between 10 p.m. and 5 a.m. for two to three nights a week

- Have been diagnosed with acanthosis nigricans (dark, thick, and velvety skin around the neck or in the armpits)

- Have been diagnosed with depression

- Have been diagnosed with hypertension or high blood pressure

- Travel frequently across more than two time zones at least every two weeks

- Typically eat dinner, a snack, or have a nightcap within 1 hour of going to bed (no matter what the food is)

- Typically sleep for less than 6 hours a night for two to three nights every week

- Your daily average step count was fewer than 5,000 steps/day during the last year. (You can get this number from your phone or from an activity tracker like a Fitbit.)

---

**PERSONALIZE YOUR DIABETES PREVENTION AND CARE**

Your diabetes risk score is unique to you. You cannot compare it to someone else's or think that you are fine if your score is barely over 5 points while someone else in your family is closer to 10. Even within the same household, different people can have very different risks for diabetes. For example, an overweight white female with no family history of diabetes may be at a lower risk than her Asian male husband with a family history of diabetes. Even if his weight is lower, he will automatically have 3 additional points (one each for being male, Asian, and having a family history of diabetes). Now, if this man also works a night shift, then the risk increases one additional point.

---

## BUT I FEEL FINE . . .

Many people are diagnosed with diabetes yet have no symptoms, or the symptoms are mild. If this is your case, that doesn't mean you can ignore your diagnosis and continue living exactly the way you have been. The problem is that diabetes is the *beginning* of the body's degeneration. The truth is that diabetes does not show up alone; it almost always brings its sinister friends.

By the time you are diagnosed with diabetes, you may already have other insidious, or silent, health conditions that result from having high blood sugar. Remember, your body likes to live within a narrow range of blood glucose, and that includes almost every cell and every nerve. So, when your blood glucose level goes up, different cells and organs may experience stress. Depending on how you are built or which genes you have that make certain organs stronger or weaker, those weaker organs may begin to show signs of degeneration and dysfunction. From there, your health can fold like a house of cards: as one organ goes awry, it affects the efficiency of another organ, and so on.

For example, the blood vessels carry blood to almost every cell in the body, and as such they are constantly exposed to the blood's sugar content. When blood sugar stays high, the blood vessels don't work as well: they can leak, stretch, or become clogged, any of which leads to their moving less blood around the body, and that is not good for the cells of the organs they are transporting that blood to use. Similarly, the nerve cells and their nerve endings infiltrate almost every cell or organ in the body, acting as conduits from the brain to control many bodily functions. When the blood glucose level becomes too high or drops too low, the nerve endings can become more sensitive, less sensitive, or even degenerate. For instance, when the nerve endings on our skin malfunction, we feel tingling, burning, pricking, or numbness.

Finally, the blood glucose directly or indirectly affects the strength of the "glue" that holds together the cells, muscles, and organs (e.g., a tooth with the gum, tendons, ligaments, and muscles). When the blood sugar level goes up, the strength of this glue weakens or the glue does not replenish well if there are muscle or joint injuries.

## YOUR DOCTOR KNOWS YOU HAVE DIABETES

If your doctor has told you that you have diabetes, he or she has made a clinical assessment as a result of one or more of the following blood tests taken during your annual physical. This is one of the most important reasons to have your health checked regularly.

All these tests sound confusing and complicated. In reality, they are relatively simple; what's complicated is your body's effort to control blood glucose. I recommend that you get at least two of these tests—fasting blood glucose and HbA1c—done during your annual health exam (you'll learn much more about this in Chapter 9).

FASTING BLOOD GLUCOSE (FBG). The magic number—100 over 100—represents 100 mg of glucose in 100 mL of blood (you may see it written on your doctor's notes as 100 mg/dL), which is the equivalent of 5 grams of sugar. One of the simplest ways to determine if blood glucose is well controlled is to measure it after at least 8 hours of fasting, using a home glucose meter or at a blood test center. A fasting blood glucose between 75 and 100 mg/dL is considered healthy. If your fasting blood glucose is more than 100 mg/dL, and certainly if it is above 126 mg/dL, then you will be told you have prediabetes or diabetes. Depending on how high your blood glucose is above 100 mg/dL, your doctor may order additional tests. Very rarely, your blood glucose may be too low (below 60 mg/dL): this is called *hypoglycemia* and causes dizziness.

ORAL GLUCOSE TOLERANCE TEST/POSTPRANDIAL GLUCOSE (PG). You can imagine that blood glucose may significantly increase after a meal. This blood test measures the body's ability to handle sugar or carbs immediately after eating. The standard method is to drink 75 grams of pure glucose dissolved in water and then measure the blood glucose 2 hours later. By this time, a healthy person can handle the rush of glucose and the blood glucose will not be dangerously high. If your PG test is more than 200 mg/dL, you will be told that you have prediabetes or diabetes.

RANDOM TEST. If you have any of the telltale signs of high blood glucose—feeling tired, frequent urination, numbness or tingling feeling in your feet—a simple blood test at a random time of the day (whether or not you fasted) can confirm your suspicions. If your random test is more than 200 mg/dL, you will be told that you have prediabetes or diabetes.

HEMOGLOBIN A1C. An indirect method of checking for diabetes is a blood test that assesses your hemoglobin A1c (HbA1c). The hemoglobin in your blood (the factor that gives blood its red color and is responsible for transporting oxygen from the lungs to the rest of the body) sticks to the glucose in the blood. If there is more blood glucose, there will be more glucose stuck to the hemoglobin. So, just by measuring how much glucose is stuck to the hemoglobin, one can figure out the average level of glucose in the blood. If your HbA1c is more than 6.5%, then you will be told that you have prediabetes or diabetes.

Roughly every three months, the body creates a new batch of hemoglobin, so an HbA1c reading provides an average level of blood glucose over the last three months.

## THE CONNECTION BETWEEN DIABETES AND OTHER DISEASES

Having high blood sugar can weaken your body's organs and make them prone to other chronic or infectious diseases. What's more, the drugs used to treat diabetes can have adverse side effects, which can impact other organs. If left untreated, any form of diabetes can lead to a range of other diseases, from high blood pressure and heart diseases to cancer and dementia.

Diabetes is just one symptom of a dysfunctional metabolic system. *Metabolism* is the chemical reactions that occur in the body to use the nutrients we eat to produce energy, make the building blocks to repair and grow cells, and eliminate waste. When our body's metabolism goes awry, it throws off the digestion and utilization of dietary fat and sugar, and we gain weight. These added pounds can affect our blood cholesterol and consequently our health in the form of metabolic diseases: obesity, diabetes, and heart disease. This trifecta can happen together or separately. Think of the obesity and heart disease as diabetes's best friends. When you have symptoms of one, the symptoms of the other conditions can slowly appear. As these diseases and their symptoms accumulate, they affect the normal function of the rest of the body. This is referred to as *metabolic syndrome*.

Your doctor uses simple criteria to test if you are on the path to metabolic syndrome. The Third Report of the National Cholesterol Education Program (NCEP) Expert Panel on Detection, Evaluation, and

Treatment of High Blood Cholesterol in Adults (Adult Treatment Panel III) defines *metabolic syndrome* as the presence of any three of the five following traits:

- Abdominal obesity
- High blood pressure
- Laboratory abnormalities of triglycerides (a type of fat in the blood)
- Low levels of high-density lipoprotein-cholesterol (HDL-C) levels
- Fasting blood glucose test showing a blood glucose level of 126 mg/dL or higher.

Diabetes is a warning, a symptom, and a crystal ball for viewing your future physical, psychological, and emotional health. Many complications of diabetes are not reversible. For example, once your nerves die and you lose the sensation of touch on your toe or skin, it rarely comes back; once you lose perfect vision from diabetes, it does not come back. To make it plain, simple, and honest, diabetes makes life miserable, renders you less productive, and provides a less enjoyable and shorter life. Here's how diabetes fuels the diseases of metabolic syndrome, as well as a host of other conditions:

HEART DISEASES AND STROKE. For the heart to function normally it needs a healthy blood supply to ensure its cells are well nourished and to maintain perfect nerve function. These factors make sure the heartbeats are rhythmic and the heart can respond to an increase or decrease in workload. Since diabetes affects blood vessels and nerve cells, it also increases the risk of heart diseases.

Similarly, our brain needs a lot of blood circulation to keep it healthy. When the whole brain, or even just one part of the brain, does not get enough blood or oxygen, a person can have a stroke, which can be lethal. According to the American Diabetes Association, 68 percent of people age 65 or older with diabetes die from some form of heart disease; 16 percent of the same population will die of a stroke.[3] Even young people with diabetes have a very high risk of having a heart attack. We also know that people who have had one heart attack are at an increased risk for another attack. In fact, the risk of having a heart attack among people with diabetes is almost the same as for those without diabetes who have already had one heart attack.

Another form of heart disease is atherosclerosis, or hardening of the arteries. This condition often precedes a heart attack or stroke. Diabetes can increase the risk of atherosclerosis. As discussed earlier, diabetes narrows the blood vessels, which slows the blood flow. Slow blood flow along with inflammation can cause atherosclerosis. Diabetes also affects the immune cells, which can contribute to atherosclerosis. All forms of diabetes make the immune cells confused, and they consider the fat deposits along the arteries to be foreign pathogens. So, the immune cells mount an inflammatory reaction to that fat deposited along clogged or narrowed blood vessels. Exercise, on the other hand, can force a faster blood flow and thereby can reverse some of the bad effects of diabetes in terms of atherosclerosis.

OBESITY. This is generally described as excessive body weight relative to height. The traditional and most widely used definition of obesity depends on the body mass index (BMI). That is, the American Medical Association defines obesity as having a BMI of 30 or higher. But obesity is more than just being overweight; it is a condition that can affect the rest of your health. It puts you at a greater risk for developing fatty liver disease, diabetes, hypertension, heart disease, and chronic kidney disease. These diseases are all related to where you store extra body fat.

As mentioned earlier, excess energy beyond what can be stored as glycogen is converted to body fat and is stored in adipose tissue, or fat cells. When the fat cells reach their full capacity, the body can store fat in cells or organs that are not designed to store it. This compromises the function of organs such as the liver, as well as the muscles and pancreas. When there is excess fat in the cells, there is less space for those cells to carry out their normal tasks of generating energy. This factor is linked to a range of diseases, from fatty liver disease and diabetes to heart disease, high blood pressure, and even cancer.

When we carry excess body fat, there is also less space for the endoplasmic reticulum (ER), or the canal system within a cell that connects to the cell membrane and then to the outside of the cell. Cells always secrete something through this canal during the daily repair cycle. But when the ER is stressed, the cell's overall repair process is hampered. Some body fat is also converted to the type of fat that causes inflammation and is released into the blood. These inflammatory fats can contribute to inflammation all over the body.

BLINDNESS. The nerves in our retinas need a good amount of blood circulation so that we can see. If even a tiny patch of the retina gets deprived of enough blood, it cannot function normally and we can lose normal vision. Therefore, when diabetes damages those small blood vessels, you can progressively lose vision.

CANCER. Type 2 diabetes is associated with increased risks for developing several cancers, including colon, postmenopausal breast, pancreatic, liver, endometrial, and bladder cancers, as well as non-Hodgkin's lymphoma.[4] With diabetes, there are many cells that cannot function properly when they are presented with high blood glucose levels. When those cells don't work properly and cannot repair themselves, then the risk of cancer increases. What's more, the immune cells that are meant to fight off cancers cannot work properly to find and kill cancer cells in a high blood glucose environment.

DEMENTIA/ALZHEIMER'S DISEASE. Narrow and damaged blood vessels in the brain can constrict blood flow, which can lead to loss of memory and dementia. In fact, dementia and/or Alzheimer's disease is often referred to as "Type 3 diabetes." Some types of dementia can be caused by an increased blood sugar level or from an occasional low blood sugar level arising from diabetes treatment.

DENTAL DISEASES. Our teeth are attached to the jawbone through connective tissues. These connective tissues are kept alive through healthy blood circulation. The nerve endings in the gum also sense injury and can repair the connective tissues. A high blood sugar level can change the rate of blood flow, the health of those nerve endings, and the molecules that serve as the glue holding the teeth to the jawbone. It's no surprise that one of the complications of diabetes, or even one of the early signs of diabetes, is loose teeth and gum disease.[5] The link between them is so strong, in fact, that if you show up at your dentist with a loose tooth, your dentist may advise you to check your blood sugar.

DEPRESSION. Diabetes and depression are two diseases that are locked in a cycle. People with uncontrolled diabetes feel like they are on a roller-coaster ride of health complications, and dealing with a chronic illness like this can take away the joy of life. At the same time, depression can lead to making poor lifestyle decisions, such as overeating or unhealthy eating, getting less exercise, and smoking—all of which are risk factors for developing diabetes.[6]

ERECTILE DYSFUNCTION. The inability to get or maintain an erection firm enough for sex is common in men who have diabetes, especially those with Type 2 diabetes. It can stem from a lack of blood flow caused by damaged nerves and damaged blood vessels.

FOOT ULCERS. Nerve cell damage can make our toes and feet numb, so if we have a bruise or cut on our foot, our brain cannot sense it, and that can result in an infected foot ulcer. Diabetes-induced damage to blood vessels also makes it difficult for the body to send enough blood supply or wound-healing agents, so bruises and cuts take longer to heal. The risk of a foot or leg amputation is increased eightfold in patients who have foot ulcers.[7]

GASTROPARESIS. Nerve cells control when and how fast the gut should move digested food along the intestine. When the nerve cells in the gut don't work well, either they fail to sense when we have digested food in the stomach or fail to squeeze the intestine to move the digested food along the tube. This can lead to nausea, bloating, vomiting, heartburn, and an overabundance of bad gut microbes growing in the stomach This condition is called *gastroparesis*.

INFECTION AND INFLAMMATION. All forms of diabetes are closely linked to disorders of the immune system. The relationship between high blood glucose and body inflammation is complicated, an area of active research. However, we do know that diabetes changes the sensitivity or susceptibility of the cells and tissue to pathogens, so that some pathogens, such as viruses and bacteria, can easily infect the body. When the immune system fails to mount the proper immune response, it allows these pathogens to survive and do more damage. What's more, an overly aggressive immune response that lasts after the pathogens are cleared can cause inflammation and other damage to the body's own cells and organs. As a result, people with diabetes are more prone to infectious diseases. To make matters worse, excessive inflammation exacerbates diabetes.

KIDNEY DISEASE. The kidneys filter out toxins from the blood. For the kidneys to function normally, the blood has to pass through the blood vessels and channel into the kidneys. Diabetes can affect the quality of the blood vessels in the kidneys, and their poor quality can result in kidney dysfunction. When this happens, the kidneys cannot filter out all the toxins from the blood, and this can slowly degenerate the kidneys, thereby requiring dialysis or a kidney transplant.

MUSCLE AND JOINT PAIN. The muscles and joints need good blood circulation and nerve function to remain operational. In addition, the glue that keeps the muscles together or attached to the bones can become damaged from increased blood sugar levels. Early signs of diabetes include a "frozen shoulder," a rotator cuff injury, or muscle weakness. Muscle and joint pain is a particularly problematic complication of diabetes, because we know that one way to control diabetes is to increase one's physical activity and exercise. But if your joints and muscles become weak or are injured easily, you may not be able to exercise enough to change the course of the disease.

SKIN DISORDERS. The skin needs constant nourishment from circulating blood in order to be healthy. Its nerve endings have to work well, and the immune system has to function properly to keep the skin free of infections, or for it to have the ability to fight off those infections. Diabetes can cause many skin complications, and some of these can be early signs of diabetes. People with diabetes are prone to skin discoloration, numbness, and frequent infections from bacterial or fungal pathogens. Some of these symptoms are more apparent in areas that are far from the heart or regions that have poor circulation, or the warm moist folds of the skin.

WOMEN'S REPRODUCTIVE HEALTH. Women are at a lower risk for diabetes compared to men of the same age. However, women with diabetes are prone to women's health issues. Reproductive dysfunction is a common but little studied complication of diabetes. Depending on the age at diagnosis of diabetes, a woman's reproductive problems can manifest early on in puberty, emerge later when fertility is desired, or occur during menopause. Other gynecological implications include polycystic ovary syndrome (PCOS), which can also lead to infertility.[8]

## DIABETES AND ITS COMPLICATIONS

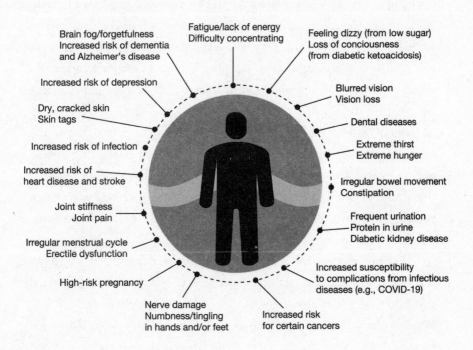

Brain fog/forgetfulness
Increased risk of dementia
and Alzheimer's disease

Fatigue/lack of energy
Difficulty concentrating

Feeling dizzy (from low sugar)
Loss of conciousness
(from diabetic ketoacidosis)

Increased risk of depression

Dry, cracked skin
Skin tags

Increased risk of infection

Increased risk of
heart disease and stroke

Joint stiffness
Joint pain

Irregular menstrual cycle
Erectile dysfunction

High-risk pregnancy

Nerve damage
Numbness/tingling
in hands and/or feet

Increased risk
for certain cancers

Blurred vision
Vision loss

Dental diseases

Extreme thirst
Extreme hunger

Irregular bowel movement
Constipation

Frequent urination
Protein in urine
Diabetic kidney disease

Increased susceptibility
to complications from infectious
diseases (e.g., COVID-19)

## CHOOSE YOUR MOTIVATION

A diagnosis of diabetes or prediabetes fundamentally threatens a basic aspiration most of us share: to live at our peak, whatever age we are. Unlike other ailments that can compromise our health for a week or two, diabetes *literally* robs us, taking away at least ten years of otherwise disease-free living.

A diagnosis of diabetes can be hard to wrap your head around. If you are in your 20s and are relatively fit, and you are told that you are prediabetic, you may go through a phase of denial, thinking there must be something wrong with the test rather than with yourself. However, I can tell you that having two "false positives" for your fasting blood glucose and your hemoglobin A1c is relatively rare. Think of it this way: if you're prediabetic, that's good news. It means that you have caught the disease early and you have time to completely reverse your diagnosis.

Take Sameer's story as a warning. During college, Sameer got into the habit of staying up very late finishing his class assignments. His hard work quickly paid off: he landed a high-paying job in the competitive software industry. For the first few years, Sameer continued with his college lifestyle: staying up late, sleeping less, and eating whatever and whenever food was available. Unfortunately, his body couldn't maintain that lifestyle without consequences, and over the next three years he gained 25 pounds, had intermittent back pain, and felt chronically tired. Sometimes he lacked mental clarity. He attributed these complaints to the stress of his job. Luckily for him, his employer required that everyone get an annual physical. When Sameer's blood work came back, his doctor told him he had prediabetes and he should lose some weight.

The "pre" part of the diagnosis made Sameer think that this news was a minor problem at best: clearly it wasn't diabetes. He also assumed that adult-onset diabetes only happened to old people in their 50s or 60s, and thought there might be a mistake in his lab results. But when he went back to see the doctor the following year, the news was worse.

This time, Sameer was told that he was now on the border, very close to full-blown Type 2 diabetes.

This doctor's message was the wake-up call Sameer needed to get himself out of denial. He started researching the implications of diabetes, and the more he learned, the less he wanted it. He had heard that one of his coworkers who had diabetes, and was also overweight, had a massive stroke in his 40s that left him paralyzed for several months. Sameer did not want to go down that same road. While researching how to manage diabetes, he came across my work and emailed me for advice. At 25, he started this same program I'm sharing with you here. In the first 12 weeks he lost some weight, and soon after that his blood sugar returned to a normal range.

If you are older, or you know that you are overweight or obese, being in denial is an even less effective strategy. The truth is, taking care of yourself isn't always easy, but if you want to have a productive life, with the ability to continue to enjoy your work and your personal interests, you have to make a change. Keep your big life goals in mind. If you can shed some weight and bring your blood sugar back down to a normal range, you can avoid diabetes and its sinister friends for a long time.

Once you cross that threshold into diabetes, however, it is difficult to focus on the parts of life that make you happiest, especially when you have to constantly worry about your health. There is a financial and emotional burden that makes it difficult to be fully present for your children or your spouse. For instance, when my daughter entered high school, one of her friends' parents was in her 40s and was already obese, diabetic, and taking multiple medications to manage her conditions. I worked with her to adopt my program, starting with increasing the number of days per week she exercised and getting better sleep. Just like every parent wants their child to graduate from high school with good grades, together we set a goal for her to have a clean bill of health by the time our children graduated from high school.

Being in your 50s or early 60s and getting diagnosed with diabetes may be more common, but it is not *normal*. In fact, it is even more dangerous than if you were diagnosed when you were younger. This is the time of life when the body goes through big changes. Sedentary men and women begin to see weight gain and a rapid loss of muscle mass that was previously protecting them from diabetes. Women go through menopause, losing the female sex hormones that also protect them from diabetes and heart diseases. These are the years when you should be planning for retirement, looking forward to the free time to travel, or starting a new hobby or finding a new passion. For many, you may also be looking forward to your children's weddings. Just like before you got married, and you wanted to lose weight to fit into that wedding dress or tuxedo, or you wanted to get fit for the active honeymoon, you need to be healthy so you can walk your children down the aisle or dance at their weddings. If you are diabetic or have developed a heart condition, foot ulcers, or joint pains, you will miss out on these special events.

What if you're a little bit older? Now you will miss out on playing with the grandkids. Dana and Brandon are a married couple in their 70s who were both diagnosed with metabolic syndrome: diabetes along with hypertension and high LDL cholesterol. They soon realized that living with metabolic syndrome is like already having had a heart attack: the risk of the second heart attack is always imminent. When they signed up for our 12-week IF program, I asked them what their motivator was. Brandon immediately said his lifelong dream has been to retire and help their daughters by babysitting their grandkids. Both of them said they had worked all their lives to save enough money, and they don't want to use that money for meeting medical expenses. They realized that if they took care of their health now, they could pass on their savings for their grandchildren's education.

## WHAT'S NEXT

Now that you understand why you've been diagnosed with prediabetes or diabetes, what's happening in your body, and what type of diabetes you may have, it's time to figure out how you can get better. The answer to that question is a lot simpler than you may imagine: it begins with aligning the way you live with your body's intended natural rhythm. I call that understanding your *circadian code*.

You often hear that diabetes and obesity are due to the lifestyle choices we make. I define "lifestyle" as the what, when, and how much you eat, sleep, move, and connect on a daily basis. But what determines a lifestyle and how best do we manage it? It boils down to timing. You know how you often juggle many different tasks by organizing them in your calendar? Similarly, your body juggles many tasks by having them occur at distinct times of the day. This is called your *circadian rhythm*. One of these tasks is keeping your blood glucose level within a healthy range during a 24-hour cycle.

When you understand your body's timing system, you will also learn to improve your daily calendar. That is, you can work with your body's preprogrammed ability to control blood glucose—that is key to mastering diabetes. What's more, the way you learn to control your blood glucose is the exact same method that can be applied to taking better care of the rest of your body, including your heart, gut, brain, and hormonal health.

## CHAPTER 2

# Broken Clocks: How Circadian Rhythms Get Out of Sync

We live on a planet with a predictable cycle of day and night, and that single constant governs everything we do. Every day, no matter where we live, all humans follow a routine that is coordinated to this cycle: we gather food and we eat it, we work, we exercise, and then we sleep. Although this cycle might seem obvious, what's really interesting is that the human species evolved to synchronize its actions to this daily rhythm, and it does so with clockwork precision. It turns out that *every task your body performs is guided by a precisely timed daily drive.* Unlocking the mystery of this daily drive is the backbone of circadian science, and it is exactly how I spend my days in my lab.

Over the past 25 years, we've learned that everything the body does is actually an intricate dance within and among the various organs, coordinated to the smallest cells that make up every body part, from the toes to the brain. Each of our cells contains the same *genome,* a hereditary data packet we received from our parents. This data packet is encoded as our DNA, and the individual segments carrying this genetic information are called *genes.* Some genes correspond to visible traits, such as hair color. Others are related to biological traits, such as blood type, risk for specific diseases like diabetes, and thousands of biochemical processes, including our circadian clock.

The health of our organs, and whether we will develop a particular illness, depends on which genes we have and how they are expressed: whether a specific gene is turned on or off, or if it is a normal gene or a mutant. For instance, some people can enjoy a wide range of food, while others complain that certain foods cause digestive discomforts like gas, bloating, or constipation. By comparing mutant genes with normal ones, we have learned a lot about how genes are supposed to work, as well as the consequences of an abnormality. Interestingly, people who can easily digest milk products have a mutation in the gene that helps break down and absorb nutrients from dairy milk; the vast majority of people around the world can't tolerate dairy.

In the field of circadian research, scientists were first able to understand how the body's internal clock works by looking for mutant organisms whose clocks ran too slow or too fast. In 1971, the California Institute of Technology fruit-fly geneticist Professor Seymour Benzer and graduate student Ron Konopka screened thousands of fruit flies, and they were able to identify three types of mutations: flies that went to sleep too early, those that went to sleep too late, or those that followed no particular pattern.[1] They also found that the offspring of those mutant fruit flies maintained the same abnormal circadian clocks as did their parents.

This initial research led scientists to understand that inside every human cell is one gene that regulates a circadian clock, which we refer to as a *period gene* (or PER gene). This period gene sends instructions to create a single protein (called PER protein), and its levels rise and fall every 24 hours. The level of PER protein informs the cell what time it is, just like we look to the position of the sun in the sky to tell us what time it is. But what makes PER protein levels rise and fall? Imagine that this protein is an ice cube that's made in your freezer. The PER gene is the ice maker that controls the exact number of ice cubes that will be made. The freezer unit makes one cube at a time and drops it into a bin under the ice maker. After a couple dozen ice cubes are in the bin, the bin becomes heavy enough and the machine turns itself off and stops making ice (likewise, the PER gene turns off once enough PER protein is made).

Every day, we take out all the ice cubes and make smoothies for the family. Then we put the bin back in the freezer, and the ice maker restarts and resumes making ice cubes until the bin is full. And because the machine's "PER gene" won't change, the number of ice cubes made every day is always the same, and the amount of time it takes for the machine to make the ice and for us to empty the ice bin is always the same. That time period is considered to be one cycle. If that cycle takes 24 hours to complete, then it is considered a circadian clock.

Yet the PER gene and its singular protein is not the only gene that controls the body's clock. In fact, we each have more than a dozen clock genes. So do mice, which makes them an ideal candidate for my research. My research team and others have systematically tested what happens when a mouse lacks one of these clock genes and how that affects its health. For instance, there is a mutation in a mouse gene called BMAL1, which completely disrupts the circadian clock and makes a mouse lose track of time. The result of this mutation is that the mouse's metabolism—the way the body breaks down food into fuel—is not right. In fact, mice that lack BMAL1 cannot control their blood glucose.

Other mutations in different mouse clock genes result in other types of abnormal metabolism. Some mice are lean yet have high blood sugar, some may have low blood sugar, some tend to eat at the wrong time and gain weight, some develop fatty liver disease, and some have weaker muscles so they cannot exercise well. Each of these mutant mice will eventually develop some of the signs of abnormal blood glucose or the symptoms/complications that usually come with diabetes. These findings have led us to believe that the major reason for having a clock within each cell is to tightly control metabolism within a healthy range. Carrying this over to humans, when your circadian clock is broken, you cannot control your metabolism and you are at risk for diabetes. This is why some of the risk factors listed in Chapter 1 (page 11) relate to how you are currently maintaining your circadian lifestyle.

## CIRCADIAN RHYTHMS FOR BRAIN AND BODY FUNCTIONS

In 2018, my team proved that up to 90 percent of all genes can be turned either on or off at different times of the day;[2] the human body simply can't have all biological functions happening at the same time.[3] Having detailed knowledge of the action of genes and their timing has given us a clear understanding of how circadian rhythm optimizes cell function. For instance:

- The nutrient or energy-sensing pathways—our cell's hunger and satiety pathways—are circadian. Just like the body feels hungry when it runs low on energy and feels satisfied after we eat, every cell in every organ has a mechanism that makes the cell hungry and opens the door to let nutrients flow in or recycles some of the stored nutrients at night while we sleep. If the cells don't open their doors to let glucose come inside after we eat a meal, then our blood sugar goes up. Aligning when we eat with when our cells are ready to soak up sugar from our food helps maintain blood glucose within a healthy range.

- The cell's metabolism pathway is circadian because the use and storage of carbohydrates, fats, and proteins is not a continuous process. When sugar is absorbed from the blood and not converted to fat or glycogen for storage and future use, the body's fat-breakdown function shuts down. Only after the most readily available sugar is depleted does the body tap into its stored fat and glycogen. This is one reason why it's so difficult to lose weight if you are eating from morning to bedtime: you are never letting your body access its stores.

- Cellular maintenance is circadian. Every chemical reaction, particularly when cells make energy for the body to use, produces a mess known as *reactive oxygen species*. This gunk is similar to kitchen grease or the oily fumes that come up from a hot pan when we are cooking. To clean up these kitchen messes, we turn on the exhaust fan and wipe up the grease after we finish cooking; similarly, cells have a timed mechanism to clean up after themselves.

- Cell repair and division is circadian. Inside and outside, cells die and need to be replaced. The replacement cells do not show up randomly; rather, the process occurs at a specific time of the day: at night, when we're asleep.

## FROM CELLS TO ORGANS

Our organs are composed of cells, and each cell secretes molecules that its neighboring cells or the whole body can use. Some molecules act like glue to keep cells together; some are chemical messengers for nearby cells or the body; and some are chemicals other cells need to repair or grow. The messenger molecules have different names. *Hormones* are "call to action" messages for specific cells to complete a specific task. For example, the hormone insulin tells a cell to open its door and take in some glucose. Another messenger is a brain chemical known as a *neurotransmitter*. For example, the neurotransmitters NPY and AgRP tell us when to feel hungry or full. The last type of messenger is called a *cytokine*, which modulates an immune reaction. Most cytokines rise and fall. If they stay high, the immune system fights against itself. This is what happens if you have an autoimmune disorder or a cytokine storm, which happens with COVID-19. If cytokine levels remain too low, then the body is prone to infection.

Every one of these molecules is released from an organ and finds its way into the bloodstream or is delivered to its neighbor. The timing of the production and secretion of these molecules is circadian, which means that every organ has its own clock that runs on a schedule best suiting its function. At the same time, every organ needs to tell other organs what it is up to, so those other organs can synchronize their efforts.

Imagine that the human body is a house and every organ is a different room, with a different clock. The clock in the bedroom reminds you when to go to sleep and wake up, the clock in the home office reminds you when you should work, and the clock in the kitchen reminds you when to eat. These internal clocks are synchronized by hormones. Just like a chain drive connects the back wheel of a bicycle to the pedals, so too the hormones are the chemical messengers synchronizing our clocks. The clock in the body's gut controls when to produce the hormones that act on the brain to signal hunger or satiety, produce digestive juices to digest food, absorb nutrition, and move waste out of the colon. The clock in the pancreas times when to produce insulin, which opens the gate in almost every cell in the body to let glucose in. And the clock in the pineal gland produces the hormone melatonin so we can go to sleep.

How do we know this? In the same 2018 study, my team began testing which of the more than 20,000 genes in the genome turn on and off at different times, in different organs. We have found that in every organ, thousands of genes turn on and off at different times, and in a synchronized fashion. For example, it takes a few genes to prepare insulin, store it in small packets, and release those packets from the pancreas. These genes turn on and off together at the same time. Similarly, a different set of genes makes sure that extra fat is broken down into smaller chunks and used to fuel the cells when the glucose supply runs low. We need these fat-burning genes to turn on and off together in order to break down body fat. In fact, we have not found any part of the body or brain that does not show the signs of a functioning circadian clock.

## THERE IS A MASTER CLOCK: THE SCN

Our internal clocks communicate between organs with the same hormonal by-products as created in the cells. And there is a small cluster of cells that function as a "master clock" in the same way as an atomic clock is a master clock for all other clocks in the world. These cells, collectively known as the *suprachiasmatic nucleus,* or SCN, are strategically located at the hypothalamus—at the center of the base of the brain, which houses the command centers for hunger, satiety, sleep, fluid balance, stress response, and more. The SCN acts as the master clock that keeps the brain and body running on time. In the evening, it tells the pineal gland to crank out the hormone melatonin so as to make us sleepy, and at the same time it tells the stress center to lower its output of stress hormone and tells the hunger center to feel less hungry. While you're sleeping, the SCN counts the hours you have slept, and a couple of hours before you wake up it tells different brain centers to prepare to wake up. In the morning, the SCN reverses the tasks, lowering production of the sleep hormone, raising the stress hormones, and sending you into the kitchen in search of food. When your SCN master clock is working well, you feel hungry at the right time and you feel sleepy at the right time; you don't feel hungry at night, you sleep just enough (not too little and not too much), your stress level goes down, and you wake up feeling energetic and ready to exercise, go to work, or go to school.

How do we know this? Well, some scientists surgically removed the SCN from a bunch of mouse brains (don't worry, it's the size of the tip of a pin, and the mouse does not die). What they found was that, without the SCN, a mouse can live a regular life; it just loses track of time. The mouse without an SCN sleeps for a few minutes before waking up, feels hungry, eats a little, feels full, walks around for a few minutes, and goes back to a few minutes of sleep—and repeats the cycle every hour. After a few days, the non-SCN mice get fat and exhibit the same telltale sign of diabetes we humans show when we have diabetes, including an elevated fasting glucose level.[4]

Although no one can come and take out a human SCN, it's pretty easy for that SCN to malfunction. Being the master clock, it needs to align with the outside world. The SCN monitors the presence or absence of light in our environment, and it shares that information with the other clocks in the brain and the body. In the morning, your SCN can tell you when to wake up (without an alarm clock) because the SCN keeps track of time and anticipates the next morning. Similarly, at the end of the day, the SCN is trying to tell you when to go to bed (around 9 or 10 p.m.) because the SCN has been keeping track of time since the morning, so it can remind your body when it's ready to go to sleep. In between, all the other organs are functioning perfectly because you're doing what you're supposed to be doing in accordance with your circadian rhythm.

Yet the truth is, you probably are not doing that. In the modern world, with our erratic lifestyles, it is difficult to maintain a fixed light–dark or day–night cycle. You may wake up way before or way after the sun comes up or go to sleep long after it has become dark. So, our SCN is almost always confused, and we may be living like those mice without an SCN—except for us, we think that's normal. When this happens, the SCN gets confused and sends the wrong timing signals to the rest of the brain and body. As a result, we may feel hungry even when our body does not need more calories (scientists use the word kilocalories or Kcal, but for simplicity, let's just call them calories), or our pancreas may not turn on to produce and release enough insulin in time for our blood sugar to be absorbed into the cells. Our stress hormones may remain high for a longer time, interfering with blood sugar. Our brain–muscle axis may get a wrong signal and we may feel lethargic or low on energy when it is daytime (you might know some people who say they are most energetic and active at night). When it comes to reversing diabetes, we want our circadian rhythm to be as closely aligned to the light–dark SCN master clock as possible.

## OUR CIRCADIAN CODE TURNS FOOD INTO ENERGY

The body needs energy every single minute of the day or night, whether we are active or asleep. If you are moderately active, your body uses energy—the equivalent of $1/10$ teaspoon sugar—every minute. But we cannot keep nibbling food or sipping juice all day and night to power our bodies—we have other things to do and we also have to sleep. So, evolution came up with a hack: a lifestyle routine that matches the rhythm of the day–night cycle. Our circadian clocks make us feel hungry during the day and less hungry at night. When your rhythms are broken, though, you may feel hungry when your body does not need to eat or you may crave to eat more than what your body needs. These broken clocks contribute to diabetes.

Our circadian rhythms carefully align the mechanisms that allow us to digest food, use it, or store and release it for later use. First, the digestive process has its own circadian rhythm by which digestive juices and acids are built up and released in the stomach and intestine during the day, and then the process slows down when we are supposed to be asleep. Digestion breaks up the *macronutrients*—carbohydrates, fat, and protein—we eat and first sends off the carbohydrates for producing the energy we immediately need. Then other circadian rhythms determine when and how much of the macronutrients are used next and where the rest are stored. For example, the liver stores the extra carbohydrates we don't need right now as glycogen and fat. After at least 12 hours of not eating, the body runs out of the readily available simple sugars and glycogen levels run low. To get the energy it needs, the body begins to break down some fat from the liver and fat tissue. These energy molecules are called *ketone bodies* and they are created in the process called *ketogenesis*. The ketone bodies provide a good source of energy for the brain and heart. In fact, animal studies have shown that when animals are hungry and have a slightly elevated level of ketone bodies, they are much better at searching for food.[5] From this finding we have learned that mild hunger does not make your brain dull; rather, it can reduce brain fog. Other ketone bodies help the immune system to fight the bacteria and pathogens that cause disease.[6]

We also have a specific set of genes in the liver that are turned on at night to break down cholesterol to make bile acid, and that bile acid travels to the gall bladder and waits there for the first bite of food, or sip of coffee, in the morning. Bile acids help the gut absorb fat, and some of that fat can travel to a special fat storage area located along the shoulders and between the shoulder blades, where it is called brown fat. When the brown fat is activated, the fat cells crank up to burn stored fat, which produces heat to keep the body warm. This might be how the body stays warm overnight.

Protein is not usually a source of energy; it is typically used to build muscles, tendons, ligaments, and skin. However, when we run low on the rest of our available energy resources, protein can be broken down to provide energy. Its smallest components are amino acids, which are used in the liver to produce glucose, which is then released into the blood to maintain blood sugar.

Our research shows that diabetes is linked to broken circadian rhythms. When a circadian rhythm is thrown off, the body cannot absorb enough sugar from the blood after we eat as quickly as it should, and the sugar remains in the blood instead of getting absorbed and processed. In some cases, the body also skips the step of burning fat and instead begins to break down protein to produce even more glucose. This results in a higher level of blood sugar, especially in the morning. And sometimes the liver forgets to stop burning protein and continues to produce glucose from protein even when we have just eaten a meal. As a result, the body gets flooded with glucose from both the food we just ate and the reserves in the liver.

Lastly, that circadian rhythm has been hardwired by our ancestral diet. Have you ever tried to hunt for food? Today it's not so hard to grab anything out of the pantry, day or night. But our bodies have developed to process food when it is most available; for our ancestors, that was during the day when they could see what they needed to hunt or gather. Similarly, at night, when it's dark, those ancestral bodies learned to rest and reset for the next day.

The foods humans eat can be broadly grouped into two types: plant based and animal based. In general, plant-based foods were easier for our ancestors to obtain. They didn't have to chase and kill vegetables, fruits, nuts, or wild corn. Plant-based food is almost always a rich source of carbohydrates; even the most protein-rich legumes or lentils are 70 percent or more carbohydrates. In contrast, animal-based foods are relatively rich in protein and fat. Although we don't have daily food records from our ancestors, we can extrapolate their food choices based on the lifestyle of a few isolated populations that still live without access to modern amenities. For people like the Bushmen of Kalahari and the Maasai of Kenya, the first foods eaten each day are made from plants and are rich in carbohydrates.[7] Ripe fruits may have enough simple sugar to be easily digested and provide instant energy. At the end of the day, they eat foods that need to be cooked: meats, tubers, vegetables, or grains. The family lights a fire, cooks the food, has a communal meal, socializes, and then goes to sleep. This pattern is how we know that the body is designed to handle carbohydrate- and sugar-rich foods early in the day. The protein, fat, and complex carbohydrate or fiber-rich foods that need cooking take longer to digest, and they provide the energy required for the long night so that we don't wake up in the middle of the night feeling hungry.

Nighttime also allows the body's recycle and repair systems to work more efficiently, as it isn't busy doing the functions needed during the day. These nighttime activities are triggered when there is less available sugar; for the body to be the most efficient at night, we need to create a sugar deficit with an overnight fast.

## DISRUPTING THE CORE CIRCADIAN RHYTHMS CAN CAUSE DIABETES

These daily rhythms of sleep, eating, and physical activity are not only a simple convenience; they are necessary to keep the body functioning well. This temporal sequence of events is programmed to run automatically, on a circadian timetable. It also requires a mechanism that anticipates what is going to happen next and can prepare the body for that imminent future. If we have a mechanism to make us tired and sleepy before our habitual bedtime, it becomes easy to fall asleep. Similarly, before we get out of a restful night of sleep, the body anticipates waking up and warms us up and pumps the heart so we get out of bed with energy. This ability of the body to anticipate what is going to happen next can be achieved only if we have an internal sense of time.

All our clocks work together like an orchestra to lay the essential foundations of health: sleep, nutrition, and activity. When the clocks work perfectly together, we have ideal health. When one rhythm is thrown off, though, the others are ultimately upset, creating a downward spiral of poor health. Unfortunately, we break those normal circadian rhythms all the time. In fact, we're so good at breaking these rhythms that some of us don't even know we had them to begin with.

## CIRCADIAN RHYTHMS AND THE THREE FOUNDATIONS OF HEALTH

**Eating**

The clocks in both the brain and body control hunger, satiety, and food choices. Clocks in the digestive system, liver, pancreas, and muscle optimize digestion, absorption, and utilization of nutrients.

**Physical activity**

There is an optimal time for daily exercise: The clocks in the brain and body control when we have the most energy and reduce the risk for injury in our muscles and joints.

**THE THREE FOUNDATIONS OF HEALTH**

**Sleep**

A circadian clock tells the brain when to sleep, how long to sleep, and informs the quality of sleep. Restorative sleep balances our mood, attention, and hormones.

## RHYTHM 1: EATING

We have found that there are two rhythms that influence eating, and they are interrelated. To find the first rhythm we asked the question: If the circadian system's main goal is to optimize energy intake, what happens when food is available at the wrong time? Once again, we turned to our mice. Typically, mice sleep during the day and prefer to be active and eat during the night. We created a simple experiment: we fed some mice only during the daytime. When the mice learned this pattern, they started waking up an hour before their food arrived to start searching for it. In other words, their brain devised a mechanism to anticipate food. Then, after eating, they went back to sleep (as they usually do during the day), and later, they strolled around at night. Their SCN, or master clock, still controlled the daily sleep–wake cycle and continued to work fine, except for a brief period during the day when they knew to wake up to eat their food.[8]

Then we looked at the rhythm of mouse liver function. We used to think that the SCN is the master clock for all rhythms and that when we eat out of sync with our SCN, then some liver genes would track the signal from the SCN and some would track food. This would confuse the liver, which may be bad for the mouse. However, we saw that almost every liver gene that turned on and off within 24 hours completely tracked the food the mice ate and ignored the signals from the SCN.[9] This new rhythm meant that the presence of food can override the SCN and reset the liver clock. This one finding completely changed how we view circadian rhythm in relation to light and food. Instead of thinking that all timing information from the outside world *has* to go through the SCN before it gets to every organ in the body, we now know that the body is able to sync with other cues. And because eating within a fixed time frame supports a robust liver clock, we can deduce that eating only within an 8- to 10-hour window—regardless of whether that window is in the morning or evening—will benefit a person more than eating throughout the entire day.

In fact, the first bite of food, or first sip of coffee, each day resets those organ clocks. In a perfect world we would wake up every day at the same time, aligning the time we eat our first meal with the time the SCN tells all our organs to start performing their tasks. This would harmonize all the clocks in our body and brain, and we would be at our best health. That first meal would be, at the earliest, 1 to 2 hours after you first wake up. However, most of us don't live our lives with clockwork precision. Even if we are mostly disciplined and consistently get 7 to 8 hours of sleep each night, most of us are not disciplined about when we eat our meals. In fact, our studies show that most people eat all day long and most of the night, with a small window of time when we don't eat in the middle of the night, often 2:00 a.m. to 4:00 a.m.[10] That is, we eat immediately after waking up and until we go to bed. The problem is that eating meals over a long period of time in the space of a 24-hour day confuses those organ clocks. Slowly, their broken rhythms will cause us to succumb to diabetes.

However, even if that sleep rhythm is constantly disrupted, maintaining a fixed window of time for eating—say, between 8 and 10 hours every day—keeps the rhythm strong enough so that most of our organ clocks are in sync, which better controls blood sugar. So, if you want to improve your health and manage your diabetes, the first rhythm you should pay attention to is *when you eat*.

Think about breakfast. Have you ever noticed that you feel hungry around the same time every morning, regardless of what and when you ate for dinner the night before? This happens because it's the SCN that sends the signal telling us when we are hungry—not the gut. At this point, the pancreas is also ready to secrete insulin, the muscles are ready to soak up some sugar, and the liver is ready to store some glycogen and make some fat, then send it off for storage. If you eat your breakfast consistently at the same time, in the morning when you feel hungry, everything will go right: your brain clock and liver clock are in sync with your day–night and eating–fasting cycles.

The second rhythm of eating is digestion. Every time we eat, even if it is just a small snack, the entire process of digestion, absorption, and metabolism begins, and that takes time to complete. Typically, it takes 5 to 6 hours to digest and absorb nutrients after a meal. This means that even if you are eating all your meals within a 10-hour window, your gut is working for 15 to 16 hours and is getting 8 to 9 hours of downtime to repair and rejuvenate. So, if you eat your last meal close to bedtime, your gut may not get any downtime at all while you are sleeping. That is, your gut is programmed to run slower at night. If your last meal is near your bedtime, the food may stay in your gut overnight before it is completely digested, causing indigestion, poor blood sugar absorption, and weight gain.

## FEED-O-GRAM

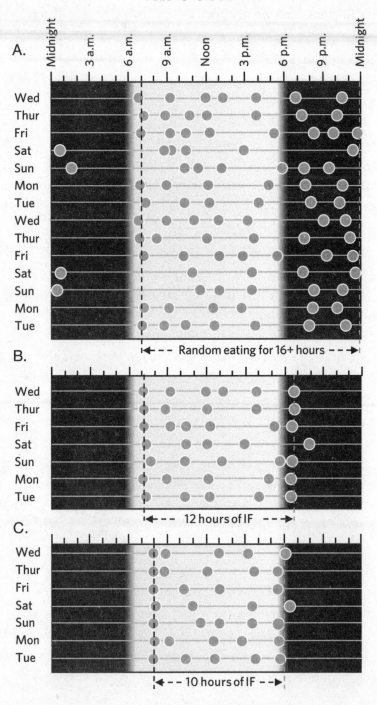

In the illustration opposite, a typical Feed-o-gram is shown for person A, who typically ate randomly from 6:00 a.m. until midnight; person B, who adopted a 12-hour IF for one week; and person C, who followed a 10-hour IF for one week. Each horizontal line represents one 24-hour day, and the position of each circle represents each time the person ate.

## RHYTHM 2: PHYSICAL ACTIVITY

When we're not eating or sleeping, we're supposed to be engaged is some form of physical activity. Our metabolism and physiology evolved so that our body can perform physical activity throughout our wakeful hours, from morning to evening. In particular, we are designed to be more active in the morning and again in the late afternoon and evening. Each of these activity windows serves a role in controlling blood glucose. The first activity window is at dawn. Outdoor exercise with exposure to the morning light, picked up by the SCN and rest of the brain, is effective in suppressing the sleep hormone melatonin, which keeps the pancreas asleep. With reduced melatonin, the early daylight primes the pancreas to produce enough insulin to take care of the glucose rush after breakfast.

In the afternoon, increasing our physical activity serves two purposes. It burns some stored glycogen from the muscles and it primes the muscles to absorb the sugar that will come from dinner. Priming the muscles is necessary because the pancreas gets tired at the end of the day and may not produce enough insulin to take care of the glucose rush that comes with an evening meal.

Physical activity can make our muscles act like a sponge, soaking up blood glucose without the help of insulin—so much so that even people with Type 1 diabetes, who do not produce insulin, can reduce the amount of insulin they need to maintain their blood glucose by being physically active. For those with Type 2 diabetes, even a 10- to 15-minute brisk walk or ride on a stationary bike after dinner is effective in reducing blood glucose to normal levels. In this sense, physical activity after a meal is almost like having an extra boost of insulin or an extra dose of diabetes medication. Compared to medicine, exercise is free and has only positive side effects.

Some people with diabetes find that exercise can increase their blood glucose levels. This can be alarming, especially if you also have an unexplained tendency to see a gradual rise in blood glucose in the morning. Those who do see an increase in blood glucose in the morning should exercise in the evening, either before or after dinner, so that they don't have such an alarming increase in blood glucose.

If you haven't been diagnosed with diabetes and you are currently mostly sedentary, any exercise at any time of the day is good. However, if you are already active and want to optimize your exercise timing, stick with late afternoon or early evening, when your muscles and joints are more flexible and therefore you have less chance of injury.

Physical activity is also the best way to spend the extra energy we gain from overeating. Although the brain uses mostly glucose as its energy source, we cannot make our brain "spend energy" by thinking extra hard. You could turn off the heater or sit outside on a cold day with no winter clothing to burn some calories to keep the body warm, but that's just not efficient. Exercising for at least an hour daily burns between 200 and 500 calories, creating an energy deficit you can count on for losing weight.

Exercise also has indirect benefits, including better sleep. As we discussed earlier, getting better sleep also reduces the craving for unhealthy food. What's more, exercise encourages the muscles to produce many biochemicals and hormones that improve the function of other organs, including the brain. Yet while we know that exercise is good for us, there is no mechanism that drives us to be physically active. To keep yourself aligned with your circadian rhythms, you have to make time to be active every day.

## RHYTHM 3: SLEEP

Sleep is the most important rhythm to maintain. We need continuous, uninterrupted sleep for 6 to 8 hours every night, and this sleep should begin and end at a consistent time. If this rhythm is disrupted, it has bad effects that reverberate throughout the brain and body. For instance, exposure to light when we should be sleeping can disrupt the SCN, which subsequently affects other rhythms in the brain and several hormone rhythms in the body. And, when your sleep rhythm is thrown off for even a few days in a row, every organ suffers. The digestive system is affected, leading to indigestion and exacerbating any digestive issues that diabetics suffer from, including gastroparesis. The heart may not work well; a 2014 study showed that one hour of sleep deprivation during the "spring forward" to Daylight Saving Time raised the risk of having a heart attack the following Monday by 24 percent, compared to other Mondays during the year.[11] The immune system may also become too reactive or too insensitive without the right amount of sleep, increasing our risk for developing an infection (and diabetics are typically more prone to infection).

Loss of sleep also makes our brain foggy, which leads to making poor health decisions. For instance, the brain actually craves sugar for energy, and poor food choices that lead to excessive sugar intake can cause the metabolism to be thrown off-balance. Studies have shown that as few as four or five nights of poor sleep (that is, sleeping 5 hours or less) can raise a person's blood glucose by several points, leading to an otherwise healthy person possibly being misdiagnosed as prediabetic.[12,13]

Reduced sleep also confuses the brain hormones that regulate hunger. The brain cannot predict how long a person is going to stay awake, and since staying awake requires more energy than sleeping, the brain increases its production of the hunger hormone. As a result, people always eat more than what is needed to stay awake for just a few extra hours. Sleep deprivation confuses the brain, making us choose unhealthy foods over healthier options. We crave energy-dense foods when we are overtired, and overeating those foods ultimately contributes to obesity and diabetes. Sleep deprivation also makes us lethargic and less active, which further contributes to excessive energy storage and leaves us with one less tool to control our blood glucose.

## IF YOU WANT TO REVERSE DIABETES, DON'T LIVE LIKE A SHIFT WORKER

When some people work the night shift, they usually try to get back to a normal routine of sleeping and eating during their off days. As you can imagine, living this way disrupts a person's circadian codes. Research has shown that overnight shift work, including the effort to get back to a "normal" schedule on off days, can increase a person's chances of developing any of several chronic diseases, including diabetes.[14]

You don't have to do real shift work to live like a shift worker, however. The general definition of shift work is staying awake for 2 to 3 hours between 10:00 p.m. and 5:00 a.m. at least once a week. So, even if you lose those 2 to 3 hours of sleep by staying awake past your usual bedtime, or by waking up earlier than your usual wake-up time, you will disrupt your rhythms much as if you were working a night shift. Similarly, any job where you are required to respond to emails, take calls, or attend to work at all hours of the day and night should be considered shift work, and includes workers in the gig economy, doctors, teachers, information technology workers, musicians, consultants, and artists.

Additionally, people who interact with others who live a few time zones away may experience similar circadian disruption. For example, if you have to wake up early or stay up late to be in a video meeting or make a phone call to your business partner, or take online classes, or visit distant loved ones a few days in a month, you are disrupting your circadian code much like a shift worker.

If your breakfast time changes by 2 or more hours on at least two days of the week, you are eating like a shift worker. Those who travel across time zones invariably are changing their eating times. Similarly, if you eat or drink late at night during the weekend, you experience the same type of circadian disruption as if you are jet-lagged. Later in this book, you'll learn how to mitigate these lifestyle disruptions.

## WHAT'S NEXT

If you are stuck in a circadian disruptive pattern, don't despair. You'll learn throughout the rest of this book how paying attention to your daily habits can be the most powerful approach to identify your circadian rhythms and return them to a normal range that keeps you healthy. We know this because healthy habits affect us on a cellular level. Our genetics have shaped our circadian rhythm, as well as a predisposition to diabetes or its complications. However, habits play a big role in our *epigenetics*, or how those genes are put into action. Although our genetic makeup is not (yet) within our control and not something we can change, there are several personal habits that we can optimize to nurture healthy circadian rhythms. In the next chapter, you'll learn why these same habits can also reverse diabetes and its related symptoms.

## CHAPTER 3

# The Circadian Breakthrough in Diabetes Research

Imagine buying a car knowing it was prone to overheating. To compensate, you pay special attention to the engine temperature and top off the coolant regularly so you don't run into trouble. In other words, you proactively treat your car's problem, and by doing so, it works perfectly. That doesn't mean that if your car has a good cooling system you don't have to maintain it. You still have to pay attention to the engine temperature because one day it might overheat anyway.

When it comes to diabetes, the same is true: regardless of predisposition and your risk factors in Chapter 1, you need to live in alignment with your circadian clocks if you want to avoid developing diabetes. In fact, we once took mutant mice that lacked a circadian clock and that had poor eating habits, and we put them on an eating program during which they ate within a fixed interval every day. We found that we could protect them completely against metabolic diseases, including diabetes.[1] In other words, a healthy eating habit can counteract the bad effects of faulty genes.

Paying attention to your health and making proactive choices that lead to good habits always pays off. My latest research shows that it is these small proactive habits that make the biggest difference in controlling, and even reversing, diabetes.

## CIRCADIAN RHYTHM RESEARCH 2.0

Over the past 20 years, research on circadian rhythm was slowly and steadily building the foundation for a deeper understanding of how the brain and body work. We knew that the clock in the brain programs us to sleep at night so that the brain can repair, cleanse, and rejuvenate so as to carry out its tasks during the day. We wanted to know if the clocks in the body's organs have similar programs.

We also knew that the clocks in those organs are programmed for better digestion, absorption, and utilization of nutrients and sugar during the day, and that these programs are hardwired and difficult to change. For example, have you ever noticed that when you eat dinner very late at night, the next day your digestion is off? You might have indigestion, bloating, constipation, or heartburn; your brain feels like you have a hangover.

It's surprising that the body has never learned to adjust to eating late at night. Even workers on a night shift who sleep during the day never entirely hack their body to fully alternate their eating routine. In fact, the longer they keep up these hours, the worse the effects.

In the last 50 years, there have been more than 200 studies regarding shift workers whose work schedules do not allow them to eat or sleep at a consistent time. Almost all these studies lead to the conclusion that shift work at night is bad for one's health—particularly, it increases the risk for diabetes. These studies looked at both men and women and were done in different countries that reflected a variety of eating styles and dietary combinations. Yet no matter where the studies were done, the results were the same: the longer someone is a night-shift worker, the higher the risk for developing diabetes.[2,3,4,5,6] This is because the body never gets used to or adjusts to living in a state that is unaligned with its circadian code.[7] And if shift workers already have diabetes, it's even harder for them to control the disease, even with medication.

Between 2000 and 2010, after the human genome was fully sequenced, scientists began to understand for the first time how our genes regulate our health. During this time, three lines of study converged, creating what was a turning point in circadian science. The first groundbreaking research in human genetics showed that some people who had either obesity or diabetes also had faulty circadian clock genes.[8] Other genetic scientists found mutations in a gene that could not perfectly process information from the sleep hormone melatonin,[9,10,11,12] which led to the discovery that melatonin influences the pancreas to release insulin after a meal is consumed.[13] A second line of research, which I was involved in, showed that mice with faulty circadian clock genes have difficulty controlling blood glucose and developed metabolic diseases.[14] Another mice study I was involved in showed that the vast majority of genes that turn on and off over a 24-hour period in the liver were involved in regulating how the liver controls sugar and fat storage.[15] This last study provided a molecular connection between the circadian clock and the regulation of blood sugar.

Taken together, these research results are nothing less than a smoking gun, akin to the discovery that cigarette smoking is bad for one's health. But we cannot stop businesses from using shift workers nor can night-shift workers hack their schedule of eating and sleeping. And, it turns out, neither can most humans. Our research that produced the Feed-o-gram in Chapter 2 (see page 40) shows that, given the opportunity, most people will eat as long as they are awake. We also know that every time we eat something, the pancreas releases insulin, which does two important jobs for metabolism: It helps absorb the sugar from the bloodstream and move it into the liver, muscle, fat, and other tissues. That insulin also signals those same organs to convert some of the sugar to body fat so that it can be accessed during times when we aren't eating. This process of sugar transportation and storage can take 2 or 3 hours after we eat. So, if we snack throughout the day and evening, the pancreas keeps producing that insulin and those organs stay in fat-making mode. In fact, eating later in the evening or into the night, when we are physically less active, further contributes to reduced energy expenditure and more fat storage. It also increases the total number of hours we eat, so the body is never directed to burn off that stored fat, as it is constantly using newly digested foods for its energy. If these habits of constant eating continue for days, weeks, months, or even years, the pancreas will eventually get stressed and not be able to produce enough insulin to meet the demand. To make matters worse, over time, the cells in the liver and other organs become so overloaded with fat that they cannot absorb the right amount of glucose from the blood, even if there is insulin available. As a result, the blood glucose levels creep up and we develop diabetes.

So, since we cannot hack the clock, how can people proactively support it for better control of the blood glucose? We believed that the answer must lie in controlling not *what* we eat but *when* we eat. And that's how the big discovery came: Living in alignment with your natural circadian rhythm is the diabetes hack we were looking for.

## A NEW THEORY FOR REVERSING DIABETES

Decades of diabetes and obesity research had led to a conclusion that a diet rich in certain types of fat or sugar causes obesity and diabetes. Over and over again, mice were fed a diet that was rich in fat and sugar, and within just 10 to 12 weeks they became obese and their blood glucose levels went up. This model became the gold-standard experiment, and has been used to help researchers understand how a poor diet and faulty genes bring us closer to diabetes, and how different drugs or good genes protect us from diabetes. Yet we thought that there must be more to the story.

We wanted to see what would happen if mice were fed an obesogenic and diabetes-promoting diet but were given all their food within a fixed window of time. We would test our hypothesis against more than 10,000 studies to interpret the results. In 2012, my laboratory took dozens of adult mice who shared the same genes, were born to the same parents, grew up in the same animal house, had the same gut bacteria (microbiome), and ate the same food. We divided these mice into two groups. Both groups ate the same high-fat and high-sugar diet, and they consumed the same number of calories every day. The only difference was that one group of mice was allowed to eat whenever they wanted (mice typically sleep during the day, so the anytime-eating mice ate one-third of their food during the day and the rest at night), and the second group was trained to eat within an 8-hour window. Within three to four days, the 8-hour mice learned the routine and ate all their food in the allotted time in order to catch up, calorie for calorie, with the unrestricted eating group. Every week, we checked how much the mice all ate and how much they weighed.

Week after week, the anytime-eating group was putting on weight, while the 8-hour eaters was barely gaining weight. At the end of four months, we tested all the mice's blood glucose levels, and there was a huge surprise. Even though both groups ate the same food and consumed the same number of calories, the anytime-eaters had higher fasting blood glucose levels, while the 8-hour eaters did not show an increase in fasting blood glucose levels. In a separate test, we found that when the anytime-eaters were given pure glucose to drink, their blood glucose shot up much higher, while the blood glucose of 8-hour eaters did not increase to the same extent.

At first, we thought something might have gone wrong with the experiment, so we repeated it in its entirety three times over the next 18 months. Every time the results came back the same: an 8-hour eating window *prevented* the development of glucose intolerance or diabetes, even with a high-carb/high-fat diet. Why? When mice eat only for 8 or 9 hours and then fast for 15 to 16 hours, their pancreas gets some rest. That is, the pancreas does not keep cranking out insulin around the clock. So, the 8-hour eaters experience low (healthy) levels of insulin in their blood during the fasting time, while the anytime-eaters have higher levels of insulin around the clock, pushing them toward diabetes.

Next, we tweaked the experiment by changing the eating window. We found that although 8-hour eaters had the most benefits, the 9- and 10-hour eaters were not too far behind. Even the 12-hour eaters reaped some (but not all) benefits. But once we went to 15 hours, we found there was no benefit at all. On the other end of the spectrum, we could not test 6- or 4-hour windows because mice cannot eat as much as their anytime-eating friends in such a short time.

Other researchers created a separate study; they tested mice with both calorie restriction and our clock research.[16] They wanted to know if a low-calorie diet was effective in reducing body weight, regardless of when the mice ate it. They fed the mice their low-calorie food at bedtime or when they first woke up. When the mice ate after they first woke up, they lost more weight than the mice who ate at bedtime. The reason was their eating pattern was aligned with their circadian code. This study implies that even if you are trying to lose weight by eating less, you may achieve more weight loss by aligning a low-calorie diet with an optimal circadian schedule. For people, this means eating most of their calories during the early part of the day instead of at night.

We also tested a wide variety of diets with different proportions of fat and sugar, including those that more closely mimicked the average diet of many people. Some of these diets caused diabetes along with weight gain, while others caused diabetes without weight gain. Irrespective of what the mice ate, we found that if they ate within a window of 8 or 9 hours, they were protected from diabetes.

We realized that eating all your food within an 8- or 9-hour period every day may not be possible or practical for everyone, week after week. So, we tested whether the mice could eat for 8 hours for five days a week and take two days off. When the mice were given two "cheat" days, they did cheat; they ate around the clock and they ate more than their 8-hour allotment. Yet, these mice were still protected from obesity and diabetes, even though they had cheated.

Next, we wanted to test mice that were already diabetic and overweight. We gave diabetic mice their regular amount and quality of food within an 8-hour period. As the weeks went by, those mice started shedding weight. And after three months, their blood glucose number substantially improved. This was truly shocking, because while some healthy habits may prevent a disease, there is not much data to show that once a disease has set in, the same healthy habit may cure or improve the condition. For example, quitting smoking may reduce the risk for lung cancer; but if an active smoker gets lung cancer, quitting smoking will not cure the cancer. Similarly, washing your hands may protect you from getting COVID-19 or flu, but once you've come down with the virus, washing your hands is not a cure. Here, we found that restricting the eating window led to a reversal of diabetes that lasts as long as the restricted eating pattern is followed.

Lastly, we wondered if this experiment would be equally successful with the "friends of diabetes." This is an important question, because diabetes is known to have many health complications. We knew that when mice eat unhealthy food (food designed to mimic the typical American diet) whenever they want to, in addition to high blood glucose, over time they develop high cholesterol and fatty liver disease, they have high levels of inflammation, and they experience growth of bad bacteria in their gut, leading to diseases of the gut. Additionally, they sleep poorly, their muscle structure is weaker, and their nerves don't work well. But we discovered that creating an 8- to 10-hour eating window worked like a silver bullet for these mice. It reduced their blood cholesterol; reduced incidence of fatty liver disease; improved overall heart condition, motor coordination, and muscle function; reduced inflammation; and improved sleep quality.

These experiments have been replicated in other labs, and the results were not much different from what we had seen in our own laboratory. In more recent studies, we found that even if the mice had disease-causing mutations, the bad effects of those bad genes could be blunted with adoption of the daily eating pattern.[17] Fun fact: both young and older mice, of both sexes, could control their blood glucose much better. So, if until now you have not paid much attention to when you eat, know that it is never too late to start.

Since our discoveries, we have "treated" hundreds of laboratory mice. These studies have provided the framework for implementing a similar strategy for people, including what benefits we can expect and whether adopting an eating window can be combined with medication or other lifestyle changes to achieve improved results. You'll learn how to apply this strategy in your life in the second half of this book.

The bottom line is that this is great news: almost every sick mouse positively responded to an eating regimen instead of eating anytime. We believe that, for people, this means that no matter what your gene pool contains, or what health conditions you may already have, you are likely to see the same positive results when you align your eating with your circadian code.

## MICE ARE NICE; HUMAN TRIALS ARE BETTER

Although our animal studies regarding diabetes were producing exciting results, media attention of our earlier research really took off. We called our eating strategy TRF (time-restricted feeding) in our mice studies, which turned into TRE (time-restricted eating) in my first book, *The Circadian Code*. Yet the popular media adopted a different label—IF, or intermittent fasting. Initially, this latter term was used to describe a 5:2 diet, whereby people are eating every other day or eating five days in a week. Now, the same term is used to describe eating all one's meals within a 6-, 8-, 10-, or 12-hour window. In fact, the most popular form of intermittent fasting is our version of time-restricted eating, so for the rest of this book we'll use the term *intermittent fasting,* or IF. However, if you want to dig deeper into the science and see our studies for yourself, Google "TRE."

Because of its popularity, thousands of people all over the world started their own experiments by creating a weight-loss diet based on intermittent fasting. Yet while we got tons of positive feedback on the internet and even in personal letters, we only heard about the good outcomes, which often offer an improved but subjective sense of how people feel when they are following the program. We didn't hear of any medically vetted quantitative measures of that improved health. And we hardly ever heard about people who found IF difficult to adopt, or about those who tried it but did not see any significant benefit. So, we wanted to understand all the possible outcomes, which is why we have to continue to do rigorous scientific studies.

In terms of diabetes, I wanted to see if we could study and document the same changes in health of people as we saw in the mice. We wanted to learn exactly *how* people adapt to intermittent fasting, what *benefits* they are likely to see, and how those benefits may *change* if they're young, old, male, female, or have a preexisting condition. Then, we wanted to explore how those benefits compare to other programs, like calorie constriction, modified diet, and medication.

The first challenge was to discover when average people eat, because if someone is already eating within an 8- to 10-hour window and has diabetes or its complications, then they are already doing IF and not benefiting from it. But if they are eating for more than 12 hours, or if that eating window changes from one day to the next and then they shorten that eating window and are more consistent, they may see benefits.

We found that more than 50 percent of adults in the United States eat over a 15-hour stretch of time or longer every day,[18] and only 10 percent eat all their food within 12 hours or less time. That means that most people eat during almost all their waking hours. In our study, 25 percent of all participants delayed their weekend breakfast by 2 hours, compared to how they ate during the week, and even this simple breakfast shift can disrupt their circadian code. But what was even more interesting was that when we asked participants when they *thought* they ate, they responded almost uniformly that they believed they ate within a 12-hour window. They weren't counting their early morning coffee with cream and sugar, or the last glass of wine or handful of nuts they'd often eat after dinner.

These findings were considered huge discoveries in the circadian and nutrition research world. There have been numerous studies of when and how much we sleep, and how it relates to our health, but until our study was done, there were few in-depth, comprehensive analyses of when people eat and how their eating patterns change from day to day. Our findings mean that almost everyone you know is eating over a long window of time and giving their body little rest from the onslaught of food every day. So, almost everyone can potentially benefit from giving their body a few more hours of rest from eating.

Another study done by a group of Harvard scientists and Spanish weight-loss nutritionists found that individuals who spread their calories over a long period of time—meaning they eat the same number of calories but eat later into the night—did not lose much weight. However, people who ate bigger meals during the day and ate little at night lost a substantial amount of weight.[19] This means that regardless of which kind of calorie-restricted diet you follow, *when* you eat is more important than what food you eat.

Next, we wanted to see if people who are eating over a longer window of time can adopt a consistent shorter window and stick to it. Indeed, we found that change is possible: people who habitually ate for 14-, 15-, or 16-hour—or even longer—windows of time can adopt an 8- to 10-hour eating window for 12 to 16 weeks. Almost everyone in our study could follow the pattern and they lost some body weight. But what was pleasantly surprising was how much they liked this new eating pattern; even a year after the study was completed, they continued to follow it. What's more, they found that they slept better, had less hunger at night, and had a better sense of energy. The same outcomes were seen in other studies around the world.

We also found that sometimes, when people reduced their eating window, they also reduced the number of calories they were eating. Our next step was to increase the rigor one notch above the level of the animal studies. My colleague Courtney Peterson, at the University of Alabama, Birmingham, recruited people without diabetes who agreed to eat their daily assigned food within a prescribed window, either eating in front of the researchers or in front of a webcam. With such a stringent study, the outcomes were clear. People who ate within a shorter window of time saw their blood glucose and blood pressure decrease, and their inflammation was also reduced. They also reported being less hungry at bedtime and felt a high level of energy throughout the day.[20]

Next, we took the experiment one step further and tested it on patients who either had elevated blood sugar or had some complications of diabetes. These patients also had metabolic syndrome: obesity, high LDL cholesterol, low HDL cholesterol, and high blood pressure. Most of them were taking either cholesterol-lowering drugs or drugs to lower their blood pressure for at least one year and had seen some improvement but had not brought their condition under control. This group had habitually eaten for 14 hours a day, or longer. They had already tried other lifestyle modifications, like eating less and exercising more, but that hadn't changed their outcome.

We ran our study for three months. The first two weeks were hard for the participants to adopt a 10-hour eating window. But after the experiment was over, the results were surprising. Almost all the participants saw some benefits in just 12 weeks. For those with high blood sugar, their levels came down. Almost all of them saw a drop in blood pressure. Those with high LDL cholesterol also saw a drop in their cholesterol. Most also had a modest weight loss.[21]

However, it turned out that the diabetes benefits were greater than what was typically expected with weight loss. While intermittent fasting may not always lead to a significant drop in body weight, it does improve several health conditions. This is important, because the finding went against previous research. Older studies showed that there were well-established formulas: any amount of weight loss (from 0 to <10%) is generally expected to result in an average blood pressure reduction of 2.675 mmHg (systolic) and 1.337 mmHg (diastolic) at 6 to 12 months.[22] Yet we found that even when people did not lose as much weight, they were still seeing benefits that were disproportionately larger than their weight loss. For example, one participant lost only 2 pounds, but her blood pressure dropped as if she had lost 5 pounds. Lastly, we also found that IF helps to manage the additional aspects of metabolic syndrome. Almost all studies on IF among overweight or obese individuals show improvements in blood pressure that meets or even exceeds the blood pressure improvement expected from medications.

## STEVE CONTROLLED DIABETES HE DIDN'T KNOW HE HAD

Steve wanted to participate in our study because he wanted to lose weight. He came to the lab weighing more than 200 pounds. It wasn't until we ran his blood work that Steve learned he was diabetic. But after 12 weeks of IF, his diabetes almost completely reversed.

During the study, we tested the participants' blood sugar levels before and after each meal. At the beginning, when Steve woke up in the morning, his blood sugar was around 130 mg/dL, and it would rise to 200 following breakfast. When we tested him during the day, following every meal, his blood sugar was going up beyond 140 mg/dL. These numbers put him firmly in the full-fledged Type 2 diabetes range. And because he had not known that he had diabetes, if Steve hadn't signed up for our trial, he would have continued with his unhealthy lifestyle, which could have further worsened his diabetes to a point where he may have ended up in the hospital.

After 12 weeks of time-restricted eating, Steve was disappointed about having lost only a modest amount of weight—only 4 percent of his body weight, or about 8 pounds. However, his morning blood sugar dropped to around 95 mg/dL, which is completely healthy, not even in the prediabetes range. And after every meal, his blood sugar barely went above 140 mg/dL, including after breakfast. And the nice thing is that he liked the IF program so much, and was so happy with the results, that he continued with the pattern when the study was over. In fact, he slowly adopted eating all his meals within a 9-hour window and continues to do so two years after the study. Steve is a great example of why IF is such good medicine: even though it is touted for weight loss, it's even more effective for diabetes and other health benefits.

## THE MANY DIABETES BENEFITS OF INTERMITTENT FASTING

Through our mice experiments we learned that being an anytime-eater is one sure way to disrupt your circadian rhythm. However, when the mice followed an IF routine, it not only reversed the disease but it also helped sustain healthier circadian clocks in all their organs. I believe that you can expect the same results when you follow an IF program, which is particularly important when you are trying to reverse or manage diabetes. In fact, our research found six different ways that IF can break the circadian diabetes code.

Intermittent fasting improves the coordination between organs and optimizes their functions. This is an important finding, because it means that when your eating routine is in alignment with your organs' clocks, the genes that are supposed to turn on and rise together in the morning do so effortlessly. For instance, when there is a strong circadian rhythm, the genes that instruct proteins to bring glucose to the cells are working in harmony with the glucose storage genes, and they rise together each time the mice ate following an IF program. This means that as glucose enters the cells, the glucose molecules are used in the right ways. As a result, blood glucose levels do not rise too high after a meal.

When insulin is produced correctly and only when needed—during the IF period and not around the clock—the fat-making genes will be at rest because they do not sense the insulin. Instead, the body turns on the fat-burning genes to create energy from our fat stores as we sleep. When the body has more time to tap into its stored glycogen during a longer overnight fast, the muscles and liver cells can use it up and make space for new glucose storage the next day. While a healthy fat cell can devote 90-plus percent of its volume to storing fat, a liver cell that has more than 20 percent of its volume as fat is a sick cell. But as the space inside all the cells becomes more available, because the fat deposits are utilized each day, the cells become healthier.

Communication between the liver and the fat-burning tissues is also enhanced with a stronger circadian code. Bile acids from the liver are another mechanism the body uses to activate the fat cells to burn more fat. In our studies, with their liver clock working as it should, the mice burned off extra fat. Not only does this improve the level of fat within the liver, but it also reduces overall cholesterol levels and lowers the risk of heart disease. However, like humans, the anytime-eating mice showed increased blood cholesterol levels. Although with an optimized liver clock, the enzyme that breaks down cholesterol into bile acids is active only for a few hours every day, when the mice could eat anytime they wanted to, their liver clock got confused and did not increase the level of cholesterol-breaking enzyme when it was needed. Yet, in the liver of the IF mice, the normal rise in cholesterol-breaking enzyme remained. Those IF mice also experienced normal blood cholesterol levels and only a slight increase in bile acids. That small increase in bile acids is considered good, as it triggers the fat cells to burn even more fat.[23] Another benefit that the IF mice received was having a warmer body temperature when they slept and were fasting, when fat-burning is at its peak. Indeed, this may be related to how our ancestors living in the wild could cope with the cold late into the night: their fat-burning systems kept them warm.

Communication between the liver and the muscles is also improved with a healthier circadian code. We learned that mice, just like us, can make glucose by breaking down protein following the instructions sent by the liver. When we fast, our muscles break down protein a little bit, releasing the protein to travel to the liver, where it is converted into glucose. But when we have diabetes, this process continues even when we eat. The extra glucose from the protein exacerbates an already flooded system. However, this didn't happen with our IF mice: their liver stayed on for only a few hours during the fasting period, and it immediately shut down when the mice ate. And since the muscle is not breaking down protein all the time to supply the extra sugar, we found that the IF mice actually gained a little bit of muscle mass. This may also happen with humans, but we don't have the data yet to prove it.

Those changes in the metabolism of glucose and fat that happened in the IF mice mirror the results of the most widely used diabetes drug, metformin. The medication tricks the body into think it is fasting and thereby helps the body absorb more glucose, burn more fat, and slow down the glucose production from protein. Hence, IF at least partly replaces what metformin is supposed to do, without the bothersome side effects of stomach upset and vitamin deficiencies.

We also know that systemic inflammation subsides with IF.[24] Systemic inflammation is the mother of many metabolic diseases, including diabetes. But the weight loss that comes with IF lessens the inflammatory fat that typically activates the immune cells causing inflammation. With less inflammation, joint pain and soreness are reduced, making it even easier to increase one's physical activity. Less fat, less cholesterol, and less inflammation mean there is less chance of developing athero-sclerosis or clogged arteries.[25] After several weeks on IF, the circadian rhythm of the autonomic nervous system resets. This autonomic nervous system controls many functions, including blood pressure regulation. In a collaborative clinical study with my colleague Dr. Pam Taub, a cardi-ologist at the University of California, San Diego, overweight patients who were at high risk for heart disease and diabetes, and who had been practicing a 10-hour IF, saw significant weight loss and reduction in fat mass, lowering their blood pressure and degree of overall inflammation. These factors all also reduced their risk for heart disease.

We also learned that IF changes the makeup of gut microbes. There is now increasing evidence that these microbes—our microbiome—affect all aspects of our health, including diabetes. When the gut has a healthy clock, it creates an environment that supports healthy gut mi-crobes and suppresses the growth of microbes that make us unhealthy. We found that IF mice showed some beneficial changes to their gut microbes, which helped them excrete more sugar in their poop. If similar changes in the gut happen in humans, it would mean that instead of ab-sorbing all the carbohydrates we eat, some may be excreted in our feces.

These six core mechanisms (see opposite) are just the beginning of our research. We cannot do the same level of in-depth studies on humans as we did on mice, as humans are much harder to control, and it would be un-ethical for researchers to take multiple samples of their liver, muscles, and fat tissues. But there are clear signs that people who do IF also reduce their excessive insulin production and their cells become more sensitive to insu-lin. The net result is that even if their pancreas is not overproducing insulin, people can still have better control of their blood glucose by following IF.

Human genetic research is the best proof we have that disruption of the circadian rhythm can increase the risk for diabetes. Over the last couple of decades, there have been many human genetic studies involv-ing diabetes. Scientists study people who have diabetes or who are obese, all done in an effort to find which genes are mutated or which genes are not working properly. These genes may not be causing the disease, but they might be a factor. It turns out that many genes that have been found to be connected with diabetes or obesity are mutations of genes that are intimately linked to our circadian rhythm. For example, one mutation in a gene that mediates the effect of melatonin turns out to be connected to obesity and diabetes. We knew that rising melatonin levels makes our brain sleepy, but it also makes our pancreas want to sleep. When we eat close to bedtime, the level of melatonin has already risen and made the pancreas slow down. This can cause the blood glucose level to stay higher for longer than we need. So, *when* we eat affects how much benefit we can gain from intermittent fasting.

There are many other genes that, when mutated, have been linked with diabetes or obesity, and a vast majority of those mutations or mutant genes turn out to be regulated by the body's clocks, with all their levels rising and falling at different times of the day. In summary, human studies have yielded strong genetic proof that there is a connection between disruption of the circadian rhythm and the development of diabetes and obesity.

SIX CORE MECHANISMS OF INTERMITTENT FASTING

THE HEALTH BENEFITS
OF INTERMITTENT FASTING

- Improved Insulin Function
- Improved Liver Function
- Increased Fat Loss
- Reduced Muscle Breakdown
- A Healthier Gut Microbiome
- Reduced Inflammation

## INTERMITTENT FASTING MAKES
## DIABETES MEDICATIONS MORE EFFICIENT

Another drug that is occasionally prescribed for controlling diabetes instead of metformin is glipizide. This class of drugs tends to increase the production of insulin and reduce blood glucose levels. If you are currently taking glipizide, consult your doctor before starting IF, because IF alone can reduce your fasting blood glucose, and when it is combined with glipizide, the fasting blood glucose may go too low. You may be able to safely reduce the drug dosage.

When you follow IF, pay attention to what time of day or night you take your medication. Some medications actually work better when they are taken in the morning or at the end of the day. Talk to your doctor to see whether your current schedule is optimizing the drug's outcome.

## WHAT'S NEXT

Now that you understand how diabetes occurs, and how disruptions to your circadian clock can make diabetes occur or worsen your chances of developing it, let's see how closely you are living in alignment with your circadian code.

## CHAPTER 4

# A Broken Circadian Rhythm Influences Diabetes

Think about what we learned about COVID-19. As an infectious disease, it has a defined cause, a set of symptoms, and specific precautions or treatments to follow to achieve a cure. But diabetes and its sinister friends are chronic conditions, so addressing them is an entirely different story. The primary cause for diabetes is not an infection; instead, it is related to our genetic predisposition and poor lifestyle choices. The key to reversing this disease—or reducing the burden of existing diabetes—lies in getting rid of bad habits and adopting better ones. The best place to start is to determine how closely you are currently aligned with an optimal circadian code.

An optimum circadian rhythm is the foundation of a good lifestyle that can help you prevent, better manage, and even reverse diabetes and its complications. This is true whether you are currently taking medication for diabetes or not. The reason is simple: diabetes medications only manage symptoms, like controlling your blood glucose levels; they do not address the underlying cause. What's more, they do nothing to control blood pressure, blood cholesterol, an unbalanced immune system, stomach diseases, and other conditions that often accompany diabetes. Each of these complications may require different drugs to bring symptoms under control. However, adopting a better circadian code addresses the underlying issues for all these symptoms and conditions. Not only can it help you prevent diabetes, or reverse early-stage diabetes, when combined with the medications you are already taking, but you will also be better able to control your diabetes and its complications.

Your lifestyle is the quality, quantity, and timing of your daily nutrition, sleep, and physical activity. We already know that we are supposed to eat healthy, get 7 to 8 hours of sleep each night, and exercise daily. If you are doing these three things with regularity, you are already ahead of the game. But if you are doing so and not optimizing your circadian code for these activities, you are missing a valuable tool. Living in alignment with your circadian code means focusing not so much on the "what" or "quality" of a healthy lifestyle as on the "when." By focusing on the when, you are harnessing the power of your circadian code, which can compensate for those times when you make less than exemplary choices in terms of quality or quantity. It is also easier to focus on when because there is only one measurement: time. And the payoff is big: by living in alignment with this internal rhythm, it will get easier to improve the quality and quantity for the rest of your lifestyle choices.

More likely than not, we are each born with a strong circadian clock that instructs every aspect of our body to work efficiently. We are at our best health when we are living at a pace that is aligned with this perfect rhythm. However, sometimes life gets in the way. It does not take too many days of disruption to completely throw off our rhythm. When we stay awake late into the night, get poor sleep, or eat continuously throughout the day, it confuses our circadian rhythms and that undermines our health.

A poor circadian code makes us vulnerable to a host of health problems. For instance, in a large study of more than 8,000 workers from 40 different organizations, researchers found that shift workers were more likely to suffer from infectious diseases, ranging from the common cold to stomach infections, than other workers.[1] These observations show us that when our rhythm is off and we come in contact with everyday bugs or viruses that we should be resistant to, or even new ones like the coronavirus, they can cause serious illness. And this research is apart from what we know about the connection between diabetes and circadian rhythms: you already learned in Chapter 2 that shift workers have a much higher rate of diabetes than the general public. This is why I say that nurturing your circadian rhythm into its optimal state acts as a grand corrector of all maladies.

You may think that having a single bad night's sleep, pulling an all-nighter at work or school, or eating a big meal late one night won't affect your blood glucose. Well, to some degree, you're right: a one-off experience is not likely to do much damage. But imagine how many times in a week or month you eat a late dinner or enjoy a bedtime snack, or how frequently you sleep less than 6 hours. Every time your circadian rhythm gets off balance, it can take two to three days for your body to readjust. That means that one day of breaking your rhythm leaves your body off balance for half the week.

It takes longer than you may imagine for your body to adjust to even the smallest glitch in your circadian rhythm. Notice how many days it takes your body to get used to the shift created by adjusting our physical clocks forward or backward just one hour for Daylight Saving Time. Now, think about shift workers, like doctors, nurses, or airline personnel. Just one night shift of work can throw off cognitive abilities for an entire week. And when we travel across time zones, we become a part-time shift worker. Cross-country travel may seem benign, but when you have to adjust to a new time zone when you arrive, you may feel jet-lagged for a few days. For most people, their circadian clock takes almost one day to adjust to each hour of time shift; for some people, it can take two days per hour of time shift. It's not just the plane travel that can be stressful for our circadian rhythms. On the day we travel, we may wake up early, cutting short our sleep time, eat earlier or later than usual, and may have difficulty falling asleep in the new place.

Similarly, when you are out late on a Friday or Saturday night, and you stay awake for three extra hours past your usual bedtime, or you delay eating breakfast by three hours on the weekend, it affects your body in the same way as flying from Los Angeles to New York. Clock scientists call this weekend habit *social jet lag*.

A change to the timing of any of the three core rhythms—sleep, eating, and activity—can be equally deleterious to your health. While a disruption does not lead directly to one specific disease, it can compromise health in many different ways. If you are already genetically susceptible to one specific type of illness, you may notice its symptoms first. For instance, if you have a sensitive stomach, circadian disruption can trigger heartburn or indigestion. If you are at risk for heart disease, circadian disruption can trigger a heart attack or stroke, as in the study I mentioned in Chapter 2.

We also know that when one rhythm goes, so go the rest. All of us have experienced this phenomenon during real or social jet lag, like when we attend a late-night party. The light you're exposed to at the party, when you would usually be sleeping, suppresses your need for sleep. Every hour you stay awake past midnight disrupts your circadian rhythm more. The next morning, you feel terrible, even if you sleep in. During the day you might find that your brain is foggy and it's harder to pay attention or make even simple decisions. Waking up late also disrupts your regular eating pattern, moving it from 8:00 a.m. to 10:00 a.m., and it may change your exercise routine. Science has shown that a sleepy brain also craves calorie-dense, unhealthy food.[2] So, even if you have been trying to eat healthy, your brain is more likely to ignore your inner voice and go for the sweet, carb-heavy breakfast you may regret later.

### THE CARLOS EXPERIMENT

One of my male colleagues at the University of California, San Diego, where I am an adjunct professor, is about 65 years old and travels at least once a month all over the country and internationally. A few months ago, when he did not show up to a meeting, I found out that he was recovering from a heart attack. I was surprised to hear the news because he always appeared to be in top health. Once he was feeling better, he told me that he had the heart attack right after returning from a trip to Europe. I suggested that we do a little experiment: we would track his heart health before and after he flew across at least one time zone. He was surprised to find that every time he traveled, either after landing in the new place or after returning to San Diego, his heartbeats were slightly outside the normal range. Now he is more careful and tries to optimize his circadian rhythm before and after travel.

## DIABETES AFFECTS YOUR CIRCADIAN CODE

It's quite possible that your state of health is linked to one or more circadian disruptions. And it's quite possible that diabetes itself, including complications or side effects related to medications that are meant to control it, may cause their own circadian disruptions. Each of these factors can cause you to sleep less or too much, change your appetite (leaving you feeling too full or too hungry), or affect your ability to engage in physical activity.

For example, obesity—one major cause of diabetes—increases the risk for obstructive sleep apnea (you'll learn more about this in Chapter 8). Not having restorative sleep because you can't breathe freely at night increases sleepiness during the day and reduces the drive to exercise. As physical activity goes down, the drive to sleep at night also reduces. This cycle keeps you awake late into the night under bright light, and when you stay awake, there's a greater likelihood that you will continue to eat late into the night. In an advance stage of diabetes, you may wake up a few times to go to the bathroom and it may be difficult to fall asleep again. Diabetes can also make your stomach bloated, or you may have acid reflux, which makes it difficult to fall asleep or may wake you up from your sleep. The cycle then continues: each of these issues not only changes the way your body controls blood glucose but can also affect other areas of your health by disrupting your circadian rhythm.

Worse, a chronic circadian disruption makes treating diabetes with medication less effective. One study found that those who are diabetic and do shift work are less likely to control their blood glucose level with medication than those who do not do shift work. In the study, 240 people already diagnosed with Type 2 diabetes were included: 120 were shift workers and 120 were day workers. The proportion of people who had good glycemic control with their medication was lower among shift workers than other workers (16% versus 28%), and the symptoms associated with hypoglycemia were more common in shift workers (43% versus 27%).[3]

---

### ARE YOU LIVING IN THE WRONG PLACE?

Professor of economics Raj Chetty has shown us that where you live influences your daily rhythms and ultimately your health and life span.[4] A neighborhood with high levels of social segregation, income inequality, accepted instability of family structure, and low-quality schools is correlated with less access to healthy foods, safe public outdoor places to exercise, and quiet places to have restful sleep. However, moving out of such a neighborhood is not always the answer. Stanford computer science professor Jure Leskovec found that people who live in cities with public transportation are more physically active, taking 2,000 to 3,000 extra steps per day.[5] When they go from home to work, they are not walking from their kitchen to the garage but, rather, from their home to the nearest bus stop or train stop—a net positive outcome.

---

## WHO IS INFLUENCING YOUR CODE?

Our habits are formed by many factors, some within our control and some seemingly beyond our control because they are influenced by others. The factors that affect your circadian clock likely fall into three buckets:

PERSONAL. Personal habits are the ones for which you have complete control. With knowledge, determination, mindfulness, and self-monitoring, you can improve your daily habits to support optimum circadian rhythms. Some of our personal habits that negatively affect a circadian code include the following behaviors, and a complete list is included in the second assessment at the end of the chapter:

- Staying indoors under dim light most of the day
- No daily physical activity/exercise/walking
- Exposure to bright light at night—working on your laptop or computer, or watching television—up until bedtime
- Having coffee, tea, caffeinated soda, dark chocolate, or chocolate desserts (like a brownie) after lunch
- Having a before-breakfast or after-dinner snack
- Stress eating, or having a snack in the middle of the night to help you fall back asleep

FAMILY OR CO-HABITING PEOPLE. The people you live with can indirectly affect your circadian rhythms. Being aware of how other people's habits can affect your own can help you manage your rhythms better. The familial habits that negatively affect your circadian code include:

- Timing your meals to accommodate someone with a different schedule; this practice is common for people with children, as parents feel compelled to share breakfast or dinner with their children, who may need a different schedule (early or late school/activities)
- Living with a shift worker
- Being a caregiver; both new mothers and caretakers for the elderly (or those with a chronic disease) often trade off a good circadian rhythm to align with the person they care for

COMMUNITY. The expectations of work (day work or shift work), as well as your community's culture, customs, and norms can affect your circadian rhythms. The community habits or workplace expectations to watch for include:

- If your work requires you to stay awake for at least 3 hours between 10:00 p.m. and 5:00 a.m. for more than 50 days a year (once a week), consider yourself a shift worker

- Working nights, early mornings, or evening shifts

- Switching from one shift to another every few days, weeks, or months

- Any job where you are required to respond to emails, take calls, or attend to work at all times of the day; the range today is almost endless and includes workers in the gig economy, doctors, teachers, information technology workers, musicians, consultants, artists, and more.

- Long working hours; cramming 12 hours into one shift (say, 6 a.m. to 6 p.m., which is normal for many day-shift nurses, retail industry employees, etc.)

- Commutes of 1 hour or more each way for work

- School schedules that begin early in the morning. Professor Horacio de la Iglesia, PhD, and I did a study on school start time changes for high school students. We found that when a school district delayed the high school start time by one hour, students got 34 minutes of extra sleep and improved their grades.[6] Although we did not add parents into the mix of participants, I assume many of them were also able to get extra sleep following the new schedule.

You can optimize your circadian code by first focusing on the factors that are personal. Then, work with your family and make decisions that are in the best interests of the group's optimal circadian alignment, such as setting a family mealtime or making small adjustments to cooking techniques that use technology to the family's advantage. For example, many IF families are using programmable pressure cookers or slow cookers to start the cooking process remotely.

You may not be able to immediately change community factors that affect your rhythm, but you can make adjustments to improve your alignment. For example, if you have a long commute or have to be at work very early in the morning, take your breakfast to go or eat dinner on your way home from work.

## WHO IS AFFECTING YOUR CIRCADIAN CODE?

**Individual/Personal Habits**

- Sleep habits
- Food preferences
- Physical activity
- Caffeine and other stimulants
- Medical conditions
- Coping strategy for stress
- Relation with digital devices
- Genes

**Family Needs/Commitments**

- Living with a shift worker
- Commitment to eat, sleep, excercise or relax with family members who may have different schedules
- Being a caregiver to a child or someone ill

**Community/Profession**

- Shift work
- Long working hours
- Long commute to work
- Public policy; e.g., school start time
- Living in an unsafe neighborhood where access to outdoor activity is limited

## TESTING YOUR CIRCADIAN CODE

First, pay attention to whether your daily sleep, activity, and eating patterns have changed over the past few months. Try to return to your normal patterns. Once you have reached what is "normal" for you, let's see if it is optimal.

I have developed two assessments that you can take in the privacy of your own home to help you see if the quality of your circadian code is affecting your health. The first one focuses on the way you think and feel right now. The second offers an opportunity for you to track how far off you are from living within an optimal rhythm.

### CIRCADIAN HEALTH ASSESSMENT #1: HOW DO YOU FEEL?

Understanding how your current health affects your circadian clock will help you make small changes that will add years of good health to your life. However, understand that there are no right or wrong answers; your mental and physical health status is as individual as you are. Don't worry if you aren't perfect; almost everyone has room for improvement. Better still, if you answer yes to any of these questions, optimizing your circadian system will only contribute to improving how you feel.

### Physical Health

The following list includes various symptoms and conditions that are related to diabetes, many of which we reviewed in Chapter 1. Any of the following can be a signal that you are edging closer to diabetes or that your existing disease is not fully under control. These symptoms or conditions can also cause a circadian disruption by affecting your sleep or eating cycles, or they may occur as a response to a poorly operating circadian code. Either way, recognizing that you have these issues, and understanding that they may be affecting you beyond the symptom itself, is the first step toward addressing them.

This is critically important, because prediabetes increases your risk for many of these health problems and reversing that trend can go a long way toward a lifetime of better health. Prediabetes can slowly and insidiously transform into Type 2 diabetes, which requires prescription medications that you will likely have to take for the rest of your life. And you may also have to cope with the adverse effects of these medications.

Place a check next to the symptom/condition if you suffer from it frequently or have received a confirmed diagnosis from a medical professional. If you haven't already, discuss these symptoms and available treatments with your doctor. These symptoms are arranged alphabetically:

☐ Abdominal pain

☐ Acanthosis nigricans (tan or brown raised areas on the sides of the neck, in the armpits and groin, on the hands, elbows, and knees)

☐ Acid reflux

☐ Allergies

☐ Asthma

☐ Athlete's foot

☐ Bacterial infections: red or swollen areas on the skin, eyelids (styes), hair follicles, or around the nails

☐ Bell's palsy

☐ Bladder infections

☐ Blisters on fingers, hands, toes, feet, legs, or forearms

☐ Bloating

☐ Boils

☐ Callouses on the feet

☐ Carpal tunnel syndrome

☐ Cataracts

☐ Change in the amount of sweat

☐ Chronic fatigue

☐ Constipation

- [ ] Decreased libido
- [ ] Dental issues: gum disease, cavities, loose teeth
- [ ] Dermopathy (light brown, scaly circular patches on the front of legs; can be mistaken for age spots)
- [ ] Diarrhea
- [ ] Difficulty adjusting from a dark room to bright light
- [ ] Difficulty breathing
- [ ] Digital sclerosis (tight, thick, waxy skin on the backs of hands, toes, and forehead)
- [ ] Disseminated granuloma annulare (a red, red-brown, or skin-colored ring or arc-shaped raised area on the fingers or ears)
- [ ] Dizziness/loss of balance/ difficulty walking
- [ ] Double vision
- [ ] Dry mouth
- [ ] Dry skin on feet
- [ ] Erectile dysfunction
- [ ] Eruptive xanthomatosis (tiny firm, yellow enlargements in the skin, each with a red halo and may itch, found on the backs of hands, feet, arms, legs, and buttocks)
- [ ] Excessive thirst
- [ ] Fainting
- [ ] Fluid retention
- [ ] Foot ulcers
- [ ] Frequent urination
- [ ] Fruity odor on breath
- [ ] Fungal infections on the skin
- [ ] Glaucoma
- [ ] Headaches
- [ ] Heart disease
- [ ] Heartburn
- [ ] High blood pressure/ hypertension
- [ ] High LDL cholesterol
- [ ] Hot flashes or disrupted sleep related to menopause
- [ ] Indigestion
- [ ] Insomnia
- [ ] Irregular menstrual cycle
- [ ] Irregular resting heartbeat
- [ ] Itching, particularly on the lower legs

- [ ] Itchy rashes in the warmer folds of the skin, including under the breasts, around nails, corners of the mouth, under the foreskin, and armpits
- [ ] Jock itch
- [ ] Joint pain
- [ ] Lower back pain
- [ ] Migraines
- [ ] Necrobiosis lipoidica diabeticorum (a dull, red, raised area that changes to a shiny scar with a violet border)
- [ ] Nephropathy (kidney disease)
- [ ] Neuropathy (tingling, pain, numbness, or weakness in your feet and hands)
- [ ] Overweight/obesity
- [ ] Pain or weakness in the legs
- [ ] Poor night vision
- [ ] Retinopathy/blurred vision
- [ ] Ringworm
- [ ] Sleep apnea
- [ ] Snoring
- [ ] Stroke
- [ ] Sweating while eating or sleeping
- [ ] Thoracic/lumbar radiculopathy (tightness of the chest or abdominal wall)
- [ ] Unilateral foot drop
- [ ] Urinary tract infections
- [ ] Vaginal dryness
- [ ] Vomiting
- [ ] Weakness/numbness on one side of the body

### Mental Health

The goal of this part of the assessment is to help you see where your mental health is affected, so that you can get yourself back into alignment with a routine that regulates insulin and enhances your circadian code. Circle the correct response if you suffer frequently.

Do you feel anxious?                                                    Y/N

Do you feel low or have frequent blue moods?              Y/N

| | |
|---|---|
| Do you struggle with attention and focus? | Y/N |
| Do you experience brain fog or poor concentration? | Y/N |
| Do you frequently lose items, like your glasses, a charging cable, or keys? | Y/N |
| Are you forgetful of names and faces? | Y/N |
| Do you rely on a calendar or to-do lists? | Y/N |
| Do you get tired in the afternoon? | Y/N |
| Do you wake feeling tired? | Y/N |
| Do you have food cravings? | Y/N |
| Do you feel like you have a lack of willpower over food? | Y/N |
| Have you been told that you are irritable? | Y/N |
| Do you have trouble making decisions? | Y/N |

If you are experiencing changes to the way you think, don't ignore that: it may be a sign that your circadian rhythm is out of whack. Without a strong circadian code, the brain does not have the right amount of time to rest and reset for the next day. One of the major functions of sleep is to detoxify our brain. It's like when you make a batch of muffins for a friend, and two out of the batch don't look quite right, so you eat those instead of putting them in the box. Similarly, the brain has to remove poorly made proteins that occurred during the daytime, and that happens in our sleep. But if our sleep is disrupted, then we cannot detoxify our brain and those toxins can build up, causing mild forms of abnormal brain function: food cravings, irritability, forgetfulness, stress, and less focus.

However, when fasting and sleeping are aligned, the brain benefits. A proper overnight fast of more than 12 hours triggers the production of hormone-like molecules in the brain called brain-derived neurotrophic factor (BDNF), which is very important for the creation of new neurons and new neuronal connections that help in terms of better memory, attention, and problem-solving capacity.

The daytime production of insulin paired with nighttime fasting is the ideal way to maintain brain health. Insulin is necessary to connect nerve cells with each other and maintain important levels of brain chemicals. But without proper insulin function, our blood sugar levels can hit extreme lows or highs, and our brain cells and neurons cannot function normally. Confusion, poor memory, and poor attention are the most likely symptoms. For example, even when you are taking diabetes medication to control your blood sugar levels, those levels may drop too low, causing hypoglycemia—this mostly occurs at night but can also happen during the day—and you correct the associated symptoms of dizziness and extreme hunger by having a glass of juice. Even corrected, the next day you may feel low energy, confused, unable to focus. On the other end of the spectrum, the same symptoms of inability to pay attention, confusion, and dizziness are signs of diabetic ketoacidosis, which occurs when your blood sugar levels get too high. If either of these conditions continues for weeks or months, that can change your brain health, causing mood disorders like feeling low, anxious, and depressed.

These symptoms can be reversed within a few hours by taking care of your diabetic ketoacidosis. However, if this condition continues, it can damage neurons and lead to a buildup of unnecessary proteins in the brain and, ultimately, Alzheimer's disease. In fact, many epidemiological studies involving more than a hundred thousand diabetic patients have shown some significant connection between people who have diabetes for many years and eventual development of dementia or Alzheimer's disease.[7] This is why some people refer to Alzheimer's as "Type 3 diabetes."

Living with chronic stress can also affect both your mental health and your insulin levels. During stressful situations—either the physical stress of doing strenuous exercise or, more often, mental stress—we produce more stress hormones, like cortisol; and having that float around in your bloodstream makes it harder for insulin to work the way it should, leading to an increase in blood sugar. Cortisol production should have a strong circadian rhythm, with peak levels reached within an hour or two of waking up in the morning,[8] so that the body can have the right energy to start the day. As the day goes on, stress can raise cortisol levels again, even though the body is not programmed to receive it. For some people with diabetes, even jogging at a moderate pace can trigger a rapid rise in cortisol and a parallel increase in blood sugar. Luckily, there is a circadian solution: by keeping to a circadian routine, you can lower stress, which also helps your body release insulin at the right levels.

---

**COMBATING STRESS WITHOUT FOOD**

Moments of mental stress may make you crave a calorie-dense snack. But because your insulin levels are already out of whack owing to the stress, eating even a small snack can raise your blood sugar much higher than if you had the same snack when you were not stressed. A better antidote is to take a 5-minute walk outside.

---

*Behavioral Habits*

Many of us do not sleep enough, eat randomly, do not participate in significant physical activity, or do our physical or mental activity at the wrong time. These personal habits can affect your circadian rhythms, as well as your risk for diabetes. To see if your daily activities are affecting your health, circle your response to the following questions.

Do you take fewer than 5,000 steps a day?                                          Y/N

Do you stay indoors under dim/fluorescent lighting
most of the day?                                                                    Y/N

Do you spend less than an hour outdoors under daylight each day? Y/N

Do you exercise after 9:00 p.m.?                                                    Y/N

Does your phone, laptop, and TV remain bright
until you fall asleep?                                                              Y/N

Do you spend more than 15 minutes in bed looking
at the computer, phone, or TV before going to sleep?                                Y/N

Do you drink or eat anything (other than water) after 7:00 p.m.?   Y/N

Do you have one or more alcoholic drinks
(cocktails, wine, or beer) after dinner?                                            Y/N

Do you have an after-dinner snack as late as
an hour before bedtime?                                                             Y/N

Do you forget to drink at least eight 8-ounce glasses
of water throughout the day?                                                        Y/N

Do you drink coffee, tea, or caffeinated soda
in the afternoon or evening?                                                        Y/N

Do you consume dark chocolates, desserts, high-carb foods
(doughnuts, pizza), or energy drinks to improve your energy level?   Y/N

Do you binge on foods regardless of hunger?                                         Y/N

Do you eat whenever food is presented to you,
even if you are not hungry?                                                         Y/N

Do you have a snack in the middle of the night
to help you fall back asleep?                                                       Y/N

Do you have a "before-breakfast" snack when you first wake up?    Y/N

Do you need a cup of coffee/tea to fully wake up?                                   Y/N

Do you sleep with a light on?                                     Y/N

Do you set aside less than 7 hours for sleep and rest every day?  Y/N

Do you need an alarm clock to wake up in the morning?            Y/N

Do you typically catch up on sleep on the weekends?              Y/N

## ASSESSING YOUR RESPONSES

It is common to have a few yes answers to these questions. In the physical and mental health sections, many of us may answer yes to one or two questions, but answering yes to three or more in each section is a sign that your circadian rhythms may not be optimal. You may also assume that some of the symptoms may be benign and negligible because many people your age or your peers may have the same symptoms. But just because these symptoms are common doesn't mean you need to live with them.

In the behavioral habits section, any yes answer is a potential disruption to your circadian clock. In our studies we have found that people typically have five or more yes answers, which means they have many different opportunities to improve their rhythm.

## CIRCADIAN HEALTH ASSESSMENT #2: TRACK YOUR DAY

The second part of the test is more of a tracking exercise. For the next week, fill out the following chart, using the descriptions as your guide. Answering these six questions for a week will give you a fair idea of your current daily rhythm. Most likely, you will find that your answers depend on many factors: whether or not you are at work, if it is a weekday or a weekend, or the unpredictability of your lifestyle. In my lab, we have monitored thousands of people all over the world, and the trend is the same: most people have different rhythms on weekdays and on weekends.

Luckily, there is an ideal circadian code for each of us, and the adjustments for individual use are not that extreme. In the second half of this book, you will learn exactly when you should be eating, sleeping, and exercising.

You may not be able to immediately incorporate every aspect of an ideal rhythm into your everyday life, but paying attention to your current rhythms will give you a good understanding of what you may be doing wrong and will help you see the places where you can make small fixes that yield big results.

In the following chapters, we'll discuss goals to work toward. But for now, let's take a brief look at the importance of each of these matters.

### When (and How) You Wake Up

When you wake up, open your eyes, and get out of bed, that first ray of bright light entering your eyes activates the melanopsin light sensors in your retina that tell your SCN that morning has arrived. Just like in a spy movie when two agents begin their mission and synchronize their watches, seeing the first ray of bright light signals the SCN to set its own clock time to the morning. Usually, when the SCN registers that you have slept enough, it will automatically nudge you to wake up—like an internal alarm clock. But if you need a real alarm clock to wake yourself up, your SCN isn't ready and still thinks it is night. This is why the goal is to be less reliant on an alarm clock and to get enough hours of sleep so that you wake up when your SCN recognizes morning.

As you fill in the chart that follows, note not only what time you woke up but also if you required an alarm clock. We don't wake up the same way our ancestors did even a century ago. In the past, when our circadian clock was in sync with the day–night cycle and we went to bed before 10:00 p.m., our SCN would wake us up around dawn. That's when you naturally stop producing melatonin and your sleep drive reduces. Dawn also brings many environmental signals to wake us up, like the first light and the seasonal noises of birds and animals. If those cues didn't do the trick, a rise in body temperature would wake you up; as melatonin levels drop to reduce the drive to sleep, the cortisol levels go up, making you feel noticeably warmer.

Today, we rarely wake up to these cues. Sleeping in a perfectly temperature-controlled bedroom with double-pane windows covered with thick curtains or blackout shades, we've all but cut out the natural morning signals of sound, light, and temperature. And when we go to sleep late, our sleep drive and melatonin levels are still high by dawn. This is why so many of us require a bone-jarring alarm clock.

### Your First Bite/Sip of the Day

Just as the first sight of light syncs your brain clock with the morning, the first bite of food signals the start of the day for the rest of the clocks in your body. In our research, we found that 80 percent of people eat or drink something other than water within an hour of waking up.[9] The next 10 percent of people have something within 2 hours, and only a small fraction of them wait for more than 2 hours to eat. Many people also reported that they often skip breakfast. These numbers just didn't add up, so we dug deeper and found out that the term *breakfast* is clearly misunderstood.

*Breakfast* means "breaking the fast": the fast is the time that passed during the night before, when you weren't eating or drinking. But what constitutes a true break in a fast? The answer is whatever triggers the stomach, liver, muscles, brain, and rest of the body to think the fast has been broken. And that encompasses "almost" anything you put in your mouth besides water.

You may think that a small cup of coffee with milk and/or sugar is not going to break a fast; most people simply associate their morning brew with an attempt to wake up the brain. Actually, as soon as we put calories in our mouth, the stomach begins to secrete gastric juice in anticipation of digesting food. Then a cascade of hormones, enzymes, and genes start their regular chores. That first cup of coffee or tea is all it takes to reset the stomach and brain clocks.

Most of our respondents consumed less than one-fourth of their total daily intake of calories between 4:00 a.m. and noon, while they ate more than 30 percent of their daily intake at night.[10] They reported that they were skipping breakfast, but in reality they were just skipping a big meal in the morning. Instead, they were eating a small snack or coffee, tea, juice, yogurt, or other items that they didn't consider a meal. However, the stomach does consider it a meal. It does not matter whether it is a cup of coffee or a whole bowl of cereal, when you break your fast, write down the time you have done so.

If you still have questions about what should count as food, just think about the day you do your fasting blood glucose test, first thing in the morning. Does your doctor tell you it is okay to drink a cup of tea or coffee before taking your blood glucose reading? Usually the answer is no.

### The End of Your Last Meal/Drink

Your brain must switch from being active to resting and rejuvenating at night, and similarly your metabolic organs need to wind down and rest for many hours. The last bite or last sip of the day signals the body to prepare to wind down, cleanse, and rejuvenate. It takes a few hours for the brain and rest of the body to get the message and start the process; it needs to be completely sure that no more calories are coming its way. So, just like a cup of coffee starts your metabolic clock, your last bite of food or drink has to be part of the digestive process for the 3 to 5 hours before the body can begin its repair and rejuvenation mode.

Culture is one of the biggest predictors of eating patterns. Although many people in the United States eat dinner early, we live in a culture of after-dinner and late-night snacking. In many Eastern countries and in parts of Europe, late-night eating is the norm; in some countries, restaurants don't even open for dinner before 9:00 p.m. And in some places, late-night dinner is the biggest meal of the day, while in others it is a small meal or leftovers from lunch.

Be honest and write down when you took your last bite or last sip (other than water and medication) of the day. You may go into this exercise thinking that you already have a schedule, but our research has shown that it is likely you don't. We use food to keep us energized or to unwind. The weekends pose a different challenge, as we are often on a completely different schedule, socializing well into the night. Keeping track of your eating will show you clearly whether you're adhering to a pattern.

### The Time You Exercise

There are distinct effects regarding the time of exercise or intense physical activity on circadian rhythm, sleep, and your blood glucose level. So, what time you exercise matters.

### The Time You Shut Off All Screens

With 24/7 social media, television, and streaming entertainment on digital devices, it becomes important to know when you are off the virtual party. You may be thinking that watching TV and being engaged in social media are ways to unwind and relax. But pay attention to whether they make you more stressed and jazzed up, which they often do.

Once we shut off our devices, the brain still takes many minutes to unwind. Our eyes receive a big share of light from those digital screens, so turning them off is also signaling that we are turning off all light input to the brain.

### The Time You Go to Sleep

Wake-up time is relatively fixed by one's work schedule, so bedtime often determines how many hours of sleep you get. Some of us have a fixed schedule during workdays. Others may have a fixed bedtime every day but wake up at different times on workdays and off days. The most accurate response is just before you shut off the lights, when you checked your last email/text/social media account, and are in bed ready to close your eyes.

## TABLE FOR ASSESSMENT #2

|  | What time did you fall asleep? | What time did you wake up? | What time did you take your first bite/sip of the day? | What time did you take your last bite/sip of the day? | What time did you exercise? | What time did you shut off all screens? |
|---|---|---|---|---|---|---|
| Monday |  |  |  |  |  |  |
| Tuesday |  |  |  |  |  |  |
| Wednesday |  |  |  |  |  |  |
| Thursday |  |  |  |  |  |  |
| Friday |  |  |  |  |  |  |
| Saturday |  |  |  |  |  |  |
| Sunday |  |  |  |  |  |  |

### Assess Your Responses

These six times will give you a good idea about your existing circadian system. There is no magic schedule that will work for everyone. However, use the following information to determine where to start making changes. The first four categories are more important and are relevant to almost everyone, whether routinely using digital screens or exercising.

- If all six times change by ±2 hours or more over the course of the week (between workdays and off days), you have a lot of room for improvement. You will easily find at least one category to fix. Sometimes fixing one category will automatically bring a few others to within an appropriate range.

- Look at the total number of hours you spend sleeping each day. The National Sleep Foundation recommends that adults get at least 7 hours a night, and that children require at least 9 hours.[11,12,13] If you are sleeping less and you wake up feeling tired in the morning, the first thing you should work on is getting to bed earlier or figuring out a schedule that allows for at least 30 more minutes of sleep in the morning. If you sleep more than 7 hours and still feel sleepy when you wake, perhaps your sleep quality is not up to mark. Remember, just three out of seven days of poor sleep will throw off your best efforts.

- Look at the total number of hours your stomach is at work. Take the earliest you eat any day of the week and the latest you eat any day of the week, ignoring only one outlier day outside your "normal" routine. That is the time period your gut is most likely staying ready to process food. If this number is more than 12, here's the good news: You have something to work on, and it will have one of the biggest impacts on your health for the rest of your life. And you're not alone. Only 10 percent of adults eat for 12 hours or less on a consistent basis without following a program such as this. People who can eat all their food within an 8- to 11-hour window most days will reap the most health benefits.

- Compare your last bite or sip time with your bedtime. The difference should ideally be 3 hours or more.

- Compare your first bite or sip time with your wake-up time. Your first bite should ideally be 1 hour or more after waking up. (In Chapter 5, I'll explain why this is so.)

---

**JOIN OUR TEAM**

My team has created an app that allows you to easily track your circadian code. Go to myCircadianClock.org to sign up to participate in a 14-week research study and get the free myCircadianClock app for your phone. It's a great way to see a more detailed look at your eating and sleeping habits. As the field of circadian rhythm progresses and we make discoveries in clinical science and public health, we will routinely transmit the new information to our users through the app and through our blog posts.

To participate, just record everything you eat and drink, including water and medicines, by simply snapping a photograph and uploading it via the app. You may also record your sleep, or you can pair an activity or sleep tracker to the app. The first two weeks of recording will help you figure out where you are with respect to your daily routines and what changes you can possibly make to address any issues.

We already have thousands of participants, and we've used their data to make some very important findings, including some of those we've mentioned in this book. As you follow the program, you can also make a big contribution to science by recording your new habits and telling us what went right and what went wrong. Your information is completely confidential and only used to help us guide you, and your experience, and will also help others.

---

## NOW THAT YOU KNOW, LET'S GET TO WORK

You may be surprised or even a little miffed that adjusting these few things is all you need to do to fix your health. What about counting calories? What about a low-carb, sugar-free, Paleo, vegan, Mediterranean, Blue Zones, Atkins, or keto diet? What about critical supplements like fish oil or green tea? You no longer have to worry about them. Just pause for a second and think—before the Industrial Revolution, people all over the world ate different types of foods depending on where they lived. There was no Chinese takeout in New York or bagels in India. Back then, diabetes was rare, instead of the norm. Yet our ancestors all had one thing in common: they ate less, did more physical activity, slept more, and completed their daily routines with clockwork precision because they did not have the luxury of light to extend the day. As I like to say, timing is everything.

In fact, timing is the grand corrector for all our behavioral habits. We have seen clinically that when people try to eat all their daily calories within 8, 10, or 12 hours, they also tap into the wisdom of the body's circadian body and brain. A natural control over calorie intake sets in, and as much as they try, they cannot actually stuff themselves with too much food in this short period of time. This means that as you get used to a smaller window of time for eating, you'll feel more satisfied with less food. This change is critical, because when you eat less and lose weight, you remove one of the major factors for developing diabetes in the first place: 80 percent of Type 2 diabetics are overweight or obese,[14] and weight loss is a primary intervention goal to improve diabetes control outside of living within your circadian code.

By focusing on timing—the *when* of your habits—you'll see that hormonal balance is restored and your immune system, mood, sleep, happiness, and libido might improve. If you are taking medications to treat your blood pressure, cholesterol, or blood sugar, fixing your circadian code may mean that you need a smaller dose to stay healthy. That's when you know you are well on your way to reversing a disease.

It takes about 12 weeks to adopt a new habit and have it affect your genes. Our existing habits and environments are like another layer of information affecting the DNA. This is called the *epigenetic code*, and it is so powerful that it reinforces our habits in a way that makes us feel like we cannot escape them. When you try to change your habits—whether it is regarding exercise or a new eating routine—the established epigenetic code makes it difficult to adopt the change as a new habit. This is when you need some willpower to fight those old habits and make new ones. As your body sees the positive results these new habits bring, it will slowly get used to them and your older epigenetic code will be replaced with a new code that will automatically nudge you to stay on your new routine.

In the next part of this book you will learn exactly when to eat, rest, play, and work so as to reverse or address diabetes. Luckily, the rest of your family can follow these patterns along with you. In this way, you can establish your family/cohabiting habits so that everyone can support one another, and ultimately all reap the benefits.

**PART II**

# Enhancing Your
# Circadian Code

## CHAPTER 5

# When to Eat

Intermittent fasting (IF) has many benefits that directly impact diabetes. As you learned in Chapter 3, by creating a longer overnight fast, IF retrains the genes and lowers the risk for developing diabetes, restores the balance between storing and burning fat, makes the natural insulin production more responsive and appropriately released, improves muscle function so that exercise becomes easier, lowers the inflammation related to diabetes, enhances the gut flora to excrete more sugar, and improves outcomes if someone is already on medication. It also addresses the ailments that show up as the sinister friends of diabetes; that is, it can reduce blood pressure to a healthy level, reduce the amount of bad cholesterol, and improve heart health.

What's more, we have found that by consolidating one's meals into a smaller window of time, it is possible to reduce one's caloric intake. That's important because if you are currently overweight, addressing your waistline is one of the best ways to start to reverse diabetes, or remove a potential risk factor for developing it in the first place. IF eating isn't necessarily considered a diet because it's never about counting calories; it is just about making you more disciplined about timing. However, we do know that when you restrict your window of opportunity, there are just so many calories one can eat in a shorter amount of time.

Our research has revolved around a 12-week program, and this is the same goal we want to set for you. It takes about 12 weeks to adopt a new habit and have it affect your genes, mitigating another potential risk factor (if your parents had diabetes, for example). What's more, this habit is an important one for reversing diabetes: the majority of our participants who completed the 12-week program found it easy to continue to practice IF by themselves for a year or more, which is what is needed in terms of controlling your health. If you want to fully reverse many forms of diabetes, you will have to stay on IF for the long haul.

One of the best things about IF is that it is so easy to start. There are just three decisions you need to make, and that's it. No special food to buy, no calorie counting, no equipment necessary, and no journaling beyond the notes you've made in Chapter 4 (unless you love to journal, then carry on!). Most other plans that reduce the risk for diabetes or aim to control diabetes are based on eating less (reduced number of calories). Calorie reduction has been tested in numerous clinical studies, and it often leads to weight loss and a reduced risk for diabetes and many other diseases that come with diabetes.[1] However, calorie reduction is hard to maintain because it is burdensome: it involves counting and recording the number of calories consumed every time you eat. And because it's so hard, people tell us all the time they feel both guilty when they cheat and deprived when they don't. IF gets you to caloric reduction almost effortlessly.

Of course, you should discuss your plans with your doctor before beginning any new eating program. If you have a fasting blood glucose of less than 100 md/dL or are prediabetic (fasting blood sugar 100–125 mg/dL) and are not on any diabetes medication, it is highly likely that you will not experience any discomfort from IF. However, in one study that combined IF and calorie restriction with patients who have Type 2 diabetes who were taking at least one medication, nearly one in three had to reduce their diabetes medications during the 12-week trial because they were experiencing nighttime hypoglycemia.[2] This, however, isn't bad news. Once you master IF, your new habit can better control your blood glucose than the medications you are currently taking. You may find that you need fewer doses of medication, or even fewer types of medication. As your doctor sees improvements and reduces your medication, you will also get the additional benefit of having fewer medication side effects.

The rest of this chapter will help you determine your "when to eat" decisions by analyzing the answers to the following questions:

- How long should your IF eating window be?
- How many meals should you eat within your window?
- What time will you start each morning?

## STEP 1: CHOOSE YOUR EATING WINDOW

If you Google the words "intermittent fasting and how many hours to fast," you will find many answers, ranging from a 16-hour fast to even a 20-hour or 22-hour fast. And you will see a bunch of variations of IF that range from reasonable to extraordinarily restrictive. The truth is, there is no definitive study on which type of fasting is sustainable for long periods of time and whether these forms of fasting are good for people with a risk for diabetes, which includes anyone who is overweight. In the clinical studies in which the effect of only 4 hours, 6 hours, or 8 hours of eating was tested on overweight or obese people, the participants were selected based on their willingness to eat within such a short window and that they did not have any of the symptoms or complications that come with diabetes. Although many of the participants could complete the 5 to 12 weeks of the study, they often complained that eating within a 4- to 6-hour window caused headaches, low energy, and nausea, and was not practical as a lifestyle.[3] In a clinical study that targeted an 8-hour eating window, some of the participants slowly drifted toward eating within 10 hours and still reaped many benefits.[4] And the other popular forms of IF have rarely reported their impact on sleep, hunger level, and energy level, all of which show desirable improvement under a 10-hour window.

Also, these more restrictive plans may not be feasible if your family does not buy in, leaving you with a completely different eating routine from the rest of those you live with. Instead, a 10-hour program, which is based on solid science, is the easiest to do and to continue for long periods of time. Our research has shown that one single, predictable, and sustained overnight fast a day is all you need to reap the many benefits of IF.

The other versions of IF that you should avoid if you are trying to reverse diabetes include the 5:2 diet. This plan has you eat normally for five days and decrease the calories consumed significantly for two days. This is the only diet connected to a study testing the impact of this IF on patients with diabetes that showed a positive effect for weight loss and fasting blood glucose.[5]

Other types of IF diets do not have backup studies but are as follows:

- Eat Stop Eat: The same routine as a 5:2 diet, but you fast completely for two days a week

- Alternate Day Fasting: Each week you fast every other day, either by not eating anything or by eating only a few hundred calories

- Warrior Diet: Every day you eat one huge meal for dinner and only small amounts of fruits and vegetables during the day

- Spontaneous Meal Skipping: You skip one or two meals when you don't feel hungry or don't have time to eat

## SET YOUR 12-WEEK SCHEDULE

Now that you understand the difference between our IF and the others, let's set some goals. While the results of maintaining a 12-hour eating window are impressive, further reducing your eating time is significantly advantageous. We have found that the best results are achieved if you can consolidate your meals to fit into a period of between 8 and 11 hours. And when it comes to weight loss, we've found the best results occur when eating within an 8- or 9-hour window, even though many will see good results starting with a 12-hour window.

In our mice studies, we found that the health benefits from eating within a 12-hour window increase when reduced to an 11-hour window and further improve with every hour dropped until an 8-hour window is achieved. Until this same study can be done with people, we can only infer that you will get better results the smaller your eating window is. Plus, holding with a shorter eating window allows for a little bit of cheating; if you follow a 10-hour IF and once in a while go to 12 hours, it's not as bad as following a 12-hour window and pushing it to 14 hours.

However, while eating for 8 hours or less may be feasible for some, or for many of us over a few days, unless you have strong willpower, it is truthfully difficult to sustain this pattern over months or years—which is what is required if you want to completely reverse diabetes or lessen your risk of developing it. Our research shows that a 10-hour eating window is sustainable, however. Additionally, you can always combine a 10-hour IF with better food choices (which you'll learn more about in the next chapter) to reach the same health benefits as come with an 8-hour IF pattern.

We've found it's best to start by establishing a 12-hour eating window for the first two weeks and then gradually reduce that to a 10-hour maintenance program. So, your IF schedule for the next 12 weeks should look like this:

**Weeks** 1–2: 12 hours of eating

**Weeks** 3–12: 10 hours of eating

---

**IT'S YOUR SCHEDULE**

Those who are not on medication and find a 10-hour fast easy, *and* do not develop any new health complications, may choose to shorten their eating window to 9 or 8 hours beginning with Week 8. You will see faster improvement with more weight loss and will improve your gut health, heart health, and focus.

If you find it difficult to maintain a 10-hour window, go back to a 12-hour IF and combine it with a healthy diet (as you'll learn about in Chapter 6).

## STEP 2: DECIDE HOW MANY MEALS TO EAT

You may have heard the recommendation to eat many small, nutritious meals spread throughout the day so as to maintain a consistent healthy blood glucose level. My personal trainer took this recommendation a step further and told me that I should eat every 2 to 4 hours up until my bedtime. While there is some merit to this idea, it was never meant for ordinary people. Instead, this eating regimen was originally devised for two extreme ends of the population.

The first group were athletes training for bodybuilding, where it was thought that eating frequent small meals was a good strategy for keeping the body in an anabolic, muscle-building mode. The second group were people with diabetes, and the recommendation was to eat small meals throughout the day to reduce the flood of sugar after each meal, so that smaller amounts of insulin could handle the rush of blood glucose. Both these ideas have been debunked in more recent studies. Read on.

The unintended consequence of the small-meals eating regimen was the creation of "healthy snacks." Based on the National Health and Nutrition Examination Survey (NHANES) data, over the past 50 years, consumption of snacks as a proportion of total calories has increased from one-tenth to one-fourth.[6] This messaging has been so powerful that when we reviewed eating patterns from the myCircadianClock app participants, we found that the traditional breakfast-lunch-dinner pattern is no longer observed, even among healthy adults. In fact, the number of eating occasions ranged from 4.2 times a day to 10.5 times a day.[7] This eating pattern is not unique to the United States, as we found a similar eating pattern in a study of adults in India.[8]

Along with more snacking, total calorie consumption has increased. One would think that added calories would be enough to end the popularity of this small-meals regimen, but many professional nutritionists and dietitians still recommend snacking. Their claim is that choosing healthy snacks can help you to meet nutrient recommendations—and feel full between meals so that you will not overeat at mealtime, thereby controlling caloric intake each day. This thinking is flawed, for many reasons:

*You don't have to feel full all the time.* Achieving a moderate level of hunger is a good sign that your stomach is ready for a meal and is tapping into your stored energy/body fat. If you cannot eat your lunch 4 to 5 hours after your breakfast, or your dinner 4 to 5 hours after your lunch, and you feel severe hunger that interferes with your thinking, it's okay to have a small snack, but only once or twice a day. Avoid snack bars, chips, pretzels, or sweetened nuts, because they are packed with calories and can cause a spike in blood sugar. Instead try roasted in-shell peanuts or pistachios. It takes time to break the shell and eat the nuts, which will slow your eating, make you mindful about what you are eating, and won't cause a spike in blood sugar. If you can't eat nuts, try a fresh fruit, vegetables like carrots or cucumber with hummus, or a cup of unsweetened yogurt.

*You can easily reach USDA nutrition recommendations in three meals.* If you have been told that you're not getting enough vitamins, fiber, or protein from your main meals, that is a warning sign that you are eating too much ultra-processed, low-quality food. Adding snacks with protein and fiber may not offset the bad effects of the rest of your diet, and certainly adds more calories.

*It's hard to keep calorie intake within a healthy range if you are constantly eating.* When you snack a few times a day, the combined calories from all those snacks can be as much as or even more than the calories in a full meal. What's more, truly healthy snacks can be hard to come by. Ultra-processed snacks, including "healthy" bars and smoothies, are everywhere; an apple, not so readily available. Or, we have a tendency to confuse hunger and thirst, and you may seek a snack when your body is really telling you to drink a glass of water. If you have the urge to snack, ask yourself when the last time was that you drank a glass of water, and try that instead.

*The recommendation to eat small meals was never meant to imply that you should do so across 16 to 18 hours a day.* Snacking after dinner is by far the worst choice you can make, and it will totally defeat any benefits you've achieved during the day. First, snacking late at night disrupts the digestive clock: you reignite your metabolism in your gut, liver, and elsewhere in your body. In this sense, you are literally waking up the body when it is meant to be slowing down, cooling down, and getting ready for sleep. Although your brain told you that you're hungry, your organs are not ready to process the food, and because your gut was not prepared to digest the food, the food won't move as fast through your digestive system as it does during the daytime. When food sits in your stomach, your stomach will secrete acid to digest the food. But if the food is not moving, this can cause acid reflux, especially if you lie down immediately after eating.

In our research, we have found that within any window of time, three meals a day is the way to go. If you eat a healthy breakfast after a long overnight fast, you may not feel hungry for the next 4 to 5 hours. Similarly, a medium-size lunch will power you for the 4 to 5 hours until dinner. This is a better schedule of eating because you are training your body to be in sync with your natural circadian code, rather than aligned with a trendy diet. Our natural circadian rhythms process for the way our ancestors ate: a few times a day, with a long overnight rest. This is important to keep in mind if you are going to be practicing IF as a family. Even if you're the only one with a risk of diabetes, the rest of the family can benefit. IF is good for everyone, at any age, to improve their sleep, focus, and physical health.

And in terms of diabetes, a clinical study has shown that people eating three (or even two) meals within a 10-hour window can better control their fasting blood glucose level than those eating three meals and three snacks. This is true even for people with insulin-dependent diabetes.[9] This study showed that for people who have been living with diabetes for more than 15 years and use insulin to manage their blood glucose, eating a healthy diet in three meals produced significantly better results than eating the same number of calories and from the same food quality in six meals spread over 12 hours or longer.

In this same study, overweight diabetic patients were limited to 1500 daily calories. Some participants were asked to eat the daily ration in three standard meals (breakfast, lunch, and dinner) and three snacks (after breakfast, afternoon snack, and bedtime snack); others were asked to eat the daily ration in three meals across 10 hours: a big breakfast (700 calories), a modest-size lunch (600 calories), and a small dinner (200 calories). After 12 weeks, the six-meal group barely lost any weight, saw no change in fasting blood glucose or hemoglobin A1c, and their insulin dosage did not change. The three-meal group saw a 5 percent drop in body weight, a reduction in fasting blood glucose and HbA1c, and were able to lower their insulin medication because they responded to that medication much better. What's more, they found that the three-meal group had a much better circadian clock. Some of their clock genes turned on at the right time and reached a higher level than the genes of those in the six-meal group. Since these clock genes regulate the breakdown and use of fat, carbohydrates, and insulin, the better clock in the three-meal group is considered to contribute to better control of diabetes.

We were not surprised with this component of the study, because circadian rhythm science had already predicted in 2014 that eating fewer meals and having a long overnight fast may give enough rest to the body to repair itself and get ready to process food more efficiently with less insulin. In another study involving people who had been living with diabetes for eight or more years, and were taking one or more medications to control their diabetes, participants were assigned to either a two-meal (breakfast and lunch) group or a six-meal (three meals and three snacks) group, with both groups eating the same number of total daily calories. After 12 weeks, the two-meal group observed more weight loss, a significant decrease in fasting blood glucose, and improvement in the body's ability to process glucose.[10]

## SET YOUR MEAL FREQUENCY

Use the information in Assessment #2 in Chapter 4 to see how often you are currently eating. Most people would say they eat three to six meals (including snacks) within a 12- to 13-hour period every day. However, we forget how often we eat late, skip or delay breakfast, or discount our snacking (a snack is anything you eat that's not a glass of water; just 1 gram of sugar can wake up your pancreas).

After you write down or use an app to track every single food or beverage you consume for at least ten days, you will discover how far from ideal your eating pattern is to support a healthy circadian rhythm.

---

**LET'S END SNACKING**

If you can figure out why you're snacking, you can create new behaviors to avoid it.

- **YOUR SLEEP-DEPRIVED BRAIN CRAVES SNACKS.** A tired brain cannot resist food, even if your body is not hungry. So, ask yourself if you are craving snacks because you did not sleep well the previous night. Maybe you need a power nap instead.

- **YOU ARE TIRED OR STRESSED IN THE MIDDLE OF THE DAY.** Late afternoon is a typical time when we start to feel a little tired. You may reach for a cup of coffee, a hot drink, or a snack to perk you up. Instead, step outside, take a deep breath, relax your muscles, or even meditate for five to ten minutes. All these behaviors can restore your energy as effectively as a snack.

- **YOU SNACK AT NIGHT.** Some people are habituated to eat a bedtime snack or drink a glass of milk before going to sleep. Remember, if you are not feeling hungry, there is no need to snack. If you feel hungry at bedtime, try just resisting the urge to snack;

after a couple of days of IF, you will notice you are less hungry at bedtime.

- **YOU HAVE NIGHTTIME HYPOGLYCEMIA.** Some people with diabetes wake up in the middle of the night feeling ravenously hungry. This occurs because their blood sugar has reached a dangerous low. They need to have a glass of juice handy to immediately bring that blood glucose up to a safe level. This is more likely to happen if you are taking diabetes medication in the evening or after dinner. Since all diabetes medications try to reduce blood glucose, and IF also reduces blood glucose, ask your doctor if you can take your diabetes medications at lunch or reduce your evening dosage. This may help you to safely practice IF without the risk of developing hypoglycemia at night. If you become hypoglycemic, always have the sugary drink your doctor has recommended.

## STEP 3: SET YOUR START TIME

The last decision you need to make is when to start your IF. The first bite of breakfast, including your first sip of coffee, tells the clocks in your gut, liver, heart, and kidneys to begin the day, so this begins your 12-hour eating window. Brushing your teeth in the morning (or at night, for that matter) will not disrupt your IF. Toothpaste doesn't count. For the first two weeks, you can eat whenever you want, as long as you stop eating exactly 12 hours after you've begun.

The question I get all the time is, "Can I choose any 12 hours I want?" The answer is that it depends. Any schedule is better than no schedule at all. However, there is an increased benefit to starting your eating window early in the day. This may be because the pancreas functions better in the first half of the day. One study found that people who delayed their lunchtime did not see the same extent of weight loss as people who ate lunch early.[11]

We've found that it's healthiest to wait and eat breakfast 1 to 2 hours after waking up. The reason is that during the early waking hours your nightly melatonin production may not have reached its daytime low yet, and your pancreas may still be asleep. At the same time, your body is experiencing the morning rise in stress hormones, which limit the function of insulin to control glucose. But within 1 to 2 hours, all your circadian rhythms are aligned and primed for a big breakfast. Your stomach is ready to digest and absorb food, your insulin production is at a healthy level, and your body is ready to process your breakfast. However, don't wait more than 4 hours, because that breakfast time will push your dinnertime too close to bedtime. When you start eating early, you are also likely to end early, at least 2 to 3 hours before going to bed. This is important, as melatonin levels begin to rise 2 to 4 hours before your average sleep time. Finishing your meals before the melatonin begins to rise is necessary so as to escape the interfering effect of melatonin on blood sugar.

Once you set your breakfast time, stick with it. The last few hours of the overnight fasting are very important. Imagine you've cleaned your house and you've put all the dirt in trash bags right by your front door. All of a sudden a wind comes and topples over the trash bags, and all your effort has been wasted. The same holds true if you eat earlier than usual in the morning. If your body isn't expecting a big flood of food to come in, all the work done overnight to cleanse your system is for naught. This is particularly important when you are on a 12-hour eating window. If you are doing a shorter eating window of, say, 8 to 10 hours, eating an earlier-than-usual breakfast once a week may not blunt the benefit too much.

You are likely to find that as you adjust to eating within a window of time, when you wake up in the morning your metabolism and hunger will demand a bigger breakfast. That's okay. Having a full breakfast fills your stomach for roughly 4 to 6 hours, making lunch at the exact midway point of a 12-hour eating window.

After breakfast, dinner is the second most important meal to align with your circadian rhythm, as it signals the end of your eating for the day. If breakfast begins at 8:00 a.m., dinner must end by 8:00 p.m. Once your body recognizes that no more food is coming, it will slowly transition to its repair and rejuvenation mode. Consider this: you don't want to lose quality family time at the end of the day, but if you have a meaningful meal for dinner, then you have that time to spend together. Our study has also shown that people who follow IF typically lose the feeling of extreme hunger that they used to have before dinnertime. And over time, they are able to reduce this meal size.

After dinner, make sure you do not lie down or go to sleep right away. I give myself 3 to 4 hours between my last bite and going to bed, which ensures better digestion and better sleep. You may feel hungry before bed, especially when you start eating within an 8- to 10-hour window. It's perfectly normal to experience these hunger pangs. You may even wake up from a deep sleep feeling hungry. Try hard to push past this by drinking a glass of water; as your body adjusts to this new rhythm, the late-night hunger will go away. And as mentioned earlier, if you are taking diabetes medication and feel extreme hunger at night along with dizziness, have the sugary drink your doctor recommends so as to combat hypoglycemia.

You'll likely find that your system gets so used to the new timing that you won't feel hungry after your target dinnertime. More surprising, people who have been on IF for a while report that if they delay their dinner too much past their target time, or have another drink or bite late at night, they can feel that the food just sits in their stomach, as if the stomach has been closed for the night and will return to work only in the morning.

## TRANSITIONING TO A 10-HOUR WINDOW

Once you've mastered the 12-hour eating window, reducing it to a 10-hour IF will be a little more challenging. At this point, we recommend that you select a 10-hour window *that works for you and your family*. Do not blindly follow someone else's advice on what worked for them or read news articles that promote skipping breakfast or skipping dinner.

The truth is you may find it difficult to follow the smaller window for more than a few days unless it somehow fits your lifestyle. So, think of an eating window that works for YOU.

To help you in finding this window, think about when you can definitely "not eat." That is, think of when you get into bed and when you typically wake up, or when you want to go to bed and want to wake up. This sleep window should be at least 8 hours (you'll learn more about this in Chapter 8). Then, subtract 2 hours from your designated bedtime. Add 1 hour to your wake-up time. You are left with a 13-hour window from which you can select your 10-hour window after Week 2.

## FIND YOUR IF WINDOW

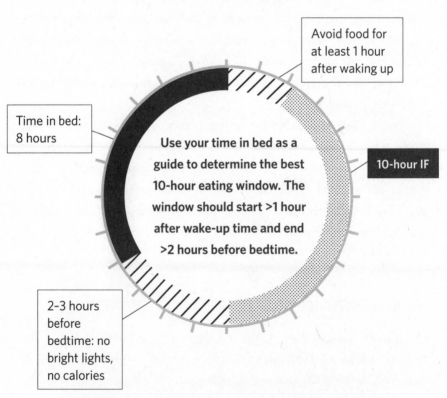

Avoid food for at least 1 hour after waking up

Time in bed: 8 hours

Use your time in bed as a guide to determine the best 10-hour eating window. The window should start >1 hour after wake-up time and end >2 hours before bedtime.

10-hour IF

2-3 hours before bedtime: no bright lights, no calories

Once you wake up, wait at least 1 hour before eating breakfast, and finish all your food and beverages for the day at least 2 hours before going to bed.

| Wake-up Time | Too Close to Wake-up Time | Ideal Eating Interval for 10-hour IF | | | Too Close to Bedtime | Bedtime |
|---|---|---|---|---|---|---|
| 4 a.m. | 5 a.m.–3 p.m. | 6 a.m.–4 p.m. | 7 a.m.–5 p.m. | 8 a.m.–6 p.m. | 9 a.m.–7 p.m. | 8 p.m. |
| 5 a.m. | 6 a.m.–4 p.m. | 7 a.m.–5 p.m. | 8 a.m.–6 p.m. | 9 a.m.–7 p.m. | 10 a.m.–8 p.m. | 9 p.m. |
| 6 a.m. | 7 a.m.–5 p.m. | 8 a.m.–6 p.m. | 9 a.m.–7 p.m. | 10 a.m.–8 p.m. | 11 a.m.–9 p.m. | 10 p.m. |
| 7 a.m. | 8 a.m.–6 p.m. | 9 a.m.–7 p.m. | 10 a.m.–8 p.m. | 11 a.m.–9 p.m. | Noon–10 p.m. | 11 p.m. |
| 8 a.m. | 9 a.m.–7 p.m. | 10 a.m.–8 p.m. | 11 a.m.–9 p.m. | Noon–10 p.m. | 1 p.m.–11 p.m. | 12 a.m. |
| 9 a.m. | 10 a.m.–8 p.m. | 11 a.m.–9 p.m. | Noon–10 p.m. | 1 p.m.–11 p.m. | 2 p.m.–midnight | 1 a.m. |
| 10 a.m. | 11 a.m.–9 p.m. | Noon–10 p.m. | 1 p.m.–11 p.m. | 2 p.m.–midnight | 3 p.m.–1 a.m. | 2 a.m. |

Use your wake-up time and bedtime to set the optimum eating window for your IF
(see white box). The gray boxes offer second-choice options, but they are either
too close to your bedtime (dark gray) or may end too late at night (light gray). Although these
windows may not be the best, they are better than eating over a longer window of time.
You can always drink plenty of water and noncaloric drinks outside the eating window.

Using the table above, you can see there are multiple 10-hour windows to choose from (and if you don't wake up on the hour, don't worry; any time within each hour is fine to start). For example, if you typically go to bed at 10:00 p.m. and get out of bed at 6:00 a.m., you might select a 10-hour window of 7:00 a.m.–5:00 p.m., or 8:00 a.m.–6:00 p.m., or 9:00 a.m.–7:00 p.m., or as late as 10:00 a.m.–8:00 p.m., or 11:00 a.m.–9:00 p.m. The 7:00 a.m.–5:00 p.m. window starts too early and is close to your wake-up time, so your breakfast may overlap with some morning melatonin. If you choose the 11:00 a.m.–9:00 p.m. window, dinner at 9:00 p.m. will be too close to your bedtime. You're now left with three possible choices: 8:00 a.m. to 6:00 p.m., or 9:00 a.m. to 7:00 p.m., or 10:00 a.m. to 8:00 p.m. There is no rigorous scientific study of which window is better. However, what we have seen from the results of the myCircadianClock app study is that people are more likely to consume alcohol, salty snacks, and sugary desserts as dinnertime moves later into the night. Therefore, if you choose an eating window that closes after 7:00 p.m., be mindful about not consuming too much alcohol, snacks, or desserts.

## THE COFFEE DILEMMA

Even if you have your morning coffee by itself, without breakfast, it still counts as the moment you break your overnight fast and open your IF eating window.

Many of us are so addicted to coffee or tea in the morning that we think we cannot survive without it. Some people need coffee or tea first thing so much so that they have coffee makers programmed to sync with their alarm clock—as soon as the alarm goes off, the coffee machine starts brewing. And once you're addicted to coffee, you may need an additional caffeine boost in the late afternoon. This second round is very likely to interfere with sleep, however. Coffee can stay in your system as long as 10 hours. That's why the conventional wisdom is to avoid coffee past noon. If you are experiencing an energy lag in the afternoon, it's possible that you're dehydrated: try a glass of water and see how you feel.

Some people ask if a tiny bit of sugar (say $1/2$ teaspoon) or a little cream or milk in the coffee or tea is a problem. Since our healthy level of fasting blood sugar should be 5 grams or less, even 2 grams of sugar is a problem, because the pancreas has to wake up to start producing insulin in order to absorb those 2 grams, and when insulin is turned on, the fat-burning genes shut down. So, it is better not to add any sugar, cream, or milk to that first cup of coffee or tea. However, keep in mind that black coffee or tea can trigger acid reflux or heartburn. If you decide to switch to black tea or coffee, you may have to reduce the amount of tea or coffee you drink so as to keep your stomach healthy.

Some people have a cup of black coffee or tea in the morning, yet don't take their first bite of food until 4 to 8 hours later. This pattern is not a perfect IF, although it may produce some benefits for people who do not have diabetes or prediabetes. However, we don't recommend this "black coffee IF" routine for people with diabetes. As your morning coffee triggers the pancreas and stomach clocks to start, the body is now primed to digest and process food. When only a little bit of food follows, you're not taking full advantage of your pancreas clock. However, a "black coffee IF" is better than no IF.

If you cannot wait until your breakfast time to have a cup of coffee or caffeinated tea, let's figure out why you need that boost:

- Some people drink coffee or tea in the morning to promote a regular bowel movement. If so, try sipping hot or warm water, or increase your fiber intake during dinner.

- If you need coffee to fully wake up, it is a good sign that you are not getting enough sleep or your sleep is not restorative. Pay attention to when you typically go to bed and try to do so earlier. You may find that after 2 or 3 weeks of the 10-hour IF, your sleep will improve and you won't feel tired in the morning.

- If you have to get to work before your eating window opens, have a small cup of black tea or black coffee to keep you awake during your commute. It is better to be caffeinated than to drive while sleepy. This is particularly important for workers who have to start an early morning shift.

## HOW TO FIX DIABETES WHILE DOING SHIFT WORK

We discussed the nature and drawbacks of various kinds of shift work in Chapter 2. There is no single, magic formula to live more healthily while doing such work. However, paying attention to a few lifestyle factors can help.

- *Alignment.* Try to be on the same shift for at least two weeks before changing to a different shift. This will help your body adapt to the new shift and recalibrate your circadian code.

- *Sleep.* Irrespective of which shift you work, shift workers in general often do not get enough sleep. Focus on increasing the number of hours in bed. Maintain a cool, dark bedroom where you can sleep whenever you can.

- *Nutrition.* Changing your diet will make a difference! Try to avoid sugary foods, alcohol, bad fats, and excessive caffeine. Then, pick an eating window that you can stick with on both workdays and off days. If you are on the night shift, try a 10- to 12-hour eating window that starts after noon and ends by midnight.

- *Exercise.* Getting enough exercise and daylight are challenges for some shift workers. Try to set aside at least 30 minutes for outdoor exercise during the day.

## CIRCADIAN TIPS FOR AIR TRAVEL OR LONG DRIVES

As I mentioned in Chapter 4, travel across time zones can wreak havoc with your circadian cycle. Here are some tips for dealing with the problems that can result.

- If you have to wake up earlier than usual on your travel day, keep your breakfast time the same. Pack a healthy breakfast and eat it at your usual breakfast time, or slightly later if you are traveling to a different time zone.

- If you are arriving at your destination past your usual dinnertime, keep your scheduled dinnertime consistent by eating this meal while you are traveling.

- For flights lasting fewer than 6 hours, it's better to skip eating on the plane and eat before boarding or after reaching your destination. You can drink water to stay hydrated during the flight.

- For eastbound flights that leave in the evening or night, you will likely arrive at your destination in the early morning. Try to stick with your regular schedule and don't stay up late binge-watching or eating. Bring earplugs or noise-canceling headsets, a neck pillow, and a sleeping mask. When you arrive at your destination, try to stay awake during the day, get some exposure to real daylight, and finish dinner by 7:00 p.m. so that you will have less trouble falling asleep.

- For westbound flights that leave during the day, you will most likely reach your destination in the late afternoon or early evening. For these flights it is okay to stay awake. But if you are sleep deprived prior to the flight, take the opportunity to catch up on sleep. Have a sleeping mask handy to help you nap better. When you arrive at your destination, you will experience a longer day than usual. That does not mean you should eat additional meals. Try not to eat on the flight: this will help you build an appetite for a post-flight early dinner at your destination.

- On the first few days you are in a new time zone, try to get the best night's sleep by using your sleeping mask, earplugs, a cool bedroom temperature (less than 68°F), and make sure the bedroom is dark.

---

**RONALD REVERSED HIS DIABETES WITH A LATER BREAKFAST**

Ronald was a participant in one of our diabetes studies. Many people would consider his lifestyle healthy: his daily eating pattern before the study involved three main meals that were spread over 14 hours. However, Ron had to be at work every day at 6:00 a.m. His routine was pretty consistent: he woke up a little after 4:00 a.m. and had breakfast at 5:00 a.m. before leaving for work. He rarely snacked, he had his lunch at 11:00 a.m., and he returned home for a home-cooked dinner by 7 p.m. He would go to bed by 9 p.m. While he knew he was overweight (he weighed 230 pounds and was only 5' 9"), he had high blood pressure, and he had high LDL cholesterol, he was shocked to find out that he also had Type 2 diabetes. His fasting blood glucose in the morning was 125 mg/dL, and throughout the day whenever he ate, his blood glucose would rise to between 180 and 200 mg/dL and stay there for several hours.

As part of the study, we told Ron to make only one change to his lifestyle: take his breakfast to work instead of eating it before he left the house and commit to eating it at 9:00 a.m. every day. While he didn't lose much weight during the 12 weeks of the study, his morning blood sugar improved to 90 mg/dL and his blood sugar levels following a meal never rose beyond 140 mg/dL. His diabetes had completely reversed. He also saw significant improvement in his blood pressure, to the extent that his doctor cut his blood pressure medication in half.

## INTERMITTENT FASTING IS A LIFESTYLE

In our mice studies, the benefits of time-restricted eating continued week after week for an entire year (which is equivalent to several years of human life) as long as the mice stayed on the schedule. In fact, the health benefits were far greater than the effect of a drug to treat the same condition. We did not change their diet and we did not reduce their number of calories consumed. Timing made the magic happen. In addition to controlling the mice's blood glucose, IF reduced their blood cholesterol, fatty liver, gut diseases, and inflammation, and even made our mice more athletic.

Can you stay on IF forever? Absolutely! As we've said, IF is not a diet. Diets are protocols people follow for short periods of time to lose weight or address a health problem. IF is a lifestyle. It is something you will want to do for the rest of your life. It is almost like brushing and flossing your teeth, where a simple routine takes care of most of your dental hygiene. The beauty of this program is that it forms the foundation for all good health. Irrespective of region, culture, or cuisine, when you and your family follow this eating program together, you will all align to a single circadian code.

You can easily stay on a 10-hour IF for most of your life. Once you start sticking to an eating window, you not only get the immediate benefits of a healthy circadian clock but you may also improve the quality and quantity of food you eat. You may see an improvement in sleep. Joint pains may reduce, making it easier to walk an extra mile or take the stairs instead of the elevator. All these changes can add up, and you will get bonus benefits.

---

### ARE YOU IN A FOOD CULT?

A food cult can be anything that combines food choices with dogma—vegan, vegetarian, low-carb/high-fat, high-carb/low-fat, low-salt, keto, Paleo, Mediterranean, and so on. Many of these diets have been shown to produce positive health benefits for those with diabetes and its complications. If you've had good results following any diet—Paleo, Atkins, ketogenic, etc.—you can combine it with a smaller window for eating. IF may in fact boost the benefits of some of these diets.

Most of the time, dieters eat fewer meals and are inadvertently doing IF anyway. If this is the case for you, you'll find IF even easier to adopt.

---

## THE TYPICAL CHALLENGES FOR INTERMITTENT FASTING

As easy as IF sounds, there are a few things you should be prepared for. The first, as I've said earlier, is to let your doctor know. Many doctors are already familiar with IF, and they can advise you as to what symptoms or complications to look out for. Set a schedule to see your doctor a few times over the 12 weeks so that he or she can adjust any medication and possibly even remove it from your daily routine. If you are taking insulin to control your diabetes, your doctor may want to follow your progress more closely. As mentioned earlier, those practicing IF may be able to reduce their insulin dose.

Next, let your family (the people you live with) know what your new eating routine will be. Decide together how you will be sharing meal-times, if everyone involved will adopt your schedule, and how you can accommodate others' schedules into your own. If someone in your family has to eat late at night or very early in the morning because of work or school, and that timing is beyond your eating window, you can still keep them company by having a sparkling water, herbal tea, or any noncaloric beverage. It's also a good idea to give others a few days to wean themselves off eating late-night snacks and breakfast as soon as they pop out of bed.

Lastly, plan where you will eat if you leave home early or get home late. If you have a long commute or you have to get to work very early in the morning, pack your breakfast and bring it to work so as to maintain your eating window. Similarly, if you come back from work very close to your bedtime, you can eat before you leave work. Then you will be having your last meal 2 to 3 hours before your bedtime. If family mealtime is important to you, switch the main meal of the day to one where you will all be together; there's no law that says dinner has to be the chosen family meal.

Once you start intermittent fasting, you'll go through a few phases during the first or second weeks. For instance, you might feel hungry when you're getting ready for bed, especially if your old routine included eating or drinking something within 3 hours of bedtime. Do not worry: it's totally normal for your stomach to crave the food it has been presented with for years. If you had a healthy dinner, that bedtime hunger will not produce dizziness and sudden loss of energy, both of which are signs of hypoglycemia. But if it does, drink what your doctor has told you to have.

Some people tell me they experience a headache during the first week or two. Since you are now eating within a 12-hour window, headaches may be due to your reduced coffee or tea consumption, or perhaps you are not drinking enough water. Try to stay hydrated. Headaches can also come from being hungry in the morning as you push forward your first meal by an hour or so. If you were used to drinking a cup of coffee or tea after waking up, try drinking a glass of warm water instead.

When you have a craving for treats or snacks within your eating window, first ask yourself "Am I hungry or thirsty?" Are you so hungry that you would readily eat raw vegetables? If not, save the snacking for another time within your eating window when you are actually hungry. If you have food cravings beyond your eating window, tell yourself you can have that snack but you just have to wait for the right time.

We have found that there is a real 6-week hurdle to this program. This is the danger zone. After six weeks, you may not yet start to see changes in your weight or blood glucose levels. If you don't see the results you're looking for, you might become disappointed or discouraged. Yet this is the exact same time when the not-so-obvious benefits begin. These benefits cannot be measured on a scale, but they may be found in better sleep, increased energy, or a reduction in systemic inflammation. Your blood levels might also be better: six weeks into the plan is a good time to get your fasting blood glucose test done to see how you are progressing.

One benefit of IF is that if you get offtrack, you can get right back on. You can still reap the benefits with an "off day" for a day or two. Let's say one Saturday night you went out with friends and blew your eating schedule. Don't panic! If your last bite of food (or drink) on Saturday night was at 11:00 p.m., you can get back on track the next day. In fact, it's quite likely that you won't feel like eating breakfast at your usual time. Listen to your body. If you're not feeling hungry, don't eat. When you finally feel hungry, go ahead and have your first meal. If that first meal is close to noon, consider it lunch. Have a well-balanced meal and then try to get back on track with your dinner. If your target is to have your dinner by 7:00 p.m., do that and go back to your original plan.

You may also find that if you are off IF for a few days or weeks, you will notice how your body does not like it. You may not sleep well, your stomach will not feel good, your energy level may decline. These are telltale signs that your body wants you to realign with IF. The good news is that once you get back on track, your body will follow, and your symptoms will disappear.

Don't beat yourself up when IF doesn't go perfectly. We're human, we make mistakes, and sometimes life really does get in the way. If you ate too much and/or too late, try one or more of the following to ease your guilt and make yourself physically more comfortable:

• Take a short walk to bring your blood glucose down. You'll learn more in Chapter 7 about the relationship between food and exercise, but in a pinch, grab your jacket and take a 15-minute stroll.

• Drink a glass of water to aid digestion.

• Plan your next meal. You may decide to delay your next morning breakfast or take a long brisk walk in the morning to get your morning hunger back.

---

**CANCELING NIGHT EATING SYNDROME**

If you have difficulty controlling your after-dinner eating, or if you wake up in the middle of the night to eat, you may be suffering from a rare medical condition called *night eating syndrome* (NES). It is generally believed that NES may result from depression, anxiety, stress, or poor results from attempts to lose weight.[12] As food consumed at night is usually made of high-glycemic carbohydrates, people with NES may suffer from being overweight.[13]

We have studied mice with NES, and we believe that there may be a genetic component. Some of our mice have a mutation in their Period 1 gene that can cause behavior similar to night eating. These mice start eating in the early afternoon (which is like 2:00 a.m. for people) and put on more weight than those who eat at their normal time. However, when these same mutant mice are allowed to eat only at night (when they are supposed to eat), their weight gain slows down.[14] This was a remarkable study, because it showed that imposing IF could counteract the bad effect of a genetic condition.

No such Period 1 mutation has been found in humans—yet. But in the coming years, we may learn more about our own genetic mutations and eating patterns. Until then, if it is impossible to hold off your urge to eat late at night, try a late IF, in which you start eating your first meal around lunchtime or even later, so that the last of your food for the day is consumed around midnight. This may not be the best approach to control NES, but it might lessen the overall effect of weight gain.

## WHAT'S NEXT

There may be some people who cannot tolerate 12 hours without food. I don't mean simply that their stomach will grumble. Stomach grumbling with hunger is a sign that the stomach is empty and is ready for business. It also means that the body is switching from using readily available energy to tapping into its stored energy. But if you feel light-headed or dizzy after 12 hours of not eating, stop the program and talk to your physician.

Sometimes people take on a challenge too intensely, such as switching from eating within a 16-hour window to a window that is only 8 hours. Or, they try to count calories and restrict their eating window at the same time. This combination can be very taxing on the body, especially if you are not used to a very low-caloric intake. Instead, I recommend that you try to start your IF with a 12-hour window without changing too much what or how much you eat. In the next chapter, you'll learn what the best foods are to reverse diabetes and make IF even easier to maintain.

## CHAPTER 6

# What to Eat

There is no doubt that *when to eat* is the most important factor when it comes to realigning your circadian code and optimizing your body to control, manage, and even reverse diabetes. But a not-so-distant second is *what to eat*. The truth is, one reason people become diabetic is that certain foods can actually control the brain and disrupt the internal clocks. However, just by making better food choices, you can retrain your body and brain so that you actually feel hunger, which signals the right time to eat your next meal and you can end the snacking/over-eating cycle. Choosing the right foods will help you stay inside your IF eating window. What's more, you can nurture your body with delicious foods from the three core nutrient groups—carbohydrates, proteins, and fats—to further optimize your code so that you are supported for all the other things you like to do each day, like exercise, sleep, and work.

The recommendations in this chapter are not your standard diet fare; in fact, I've timed out what you should eat when, so that you can turn each meal into a nutritional opportunity.

## HOW YOUR BODY USES FOOD FOR FUEL

If you want to take good care of your car so that it lasts you at least 239,000 miles (the distance between the earth and the moon), you should know some basic facts about how your car works. Similarly, if you want to stay healthy, a little bit of knowledge about how the body uses nutrition will go a long way. The bottom line is this: a balanced diet that combines the right carbs, fat, and protein is important to nourish all of your body's organs. Making the wrong food choices, particularly the wrong carbohydrates in the wrong amounts, can break this balance and disrupt the normal functioning of brain and body.

Let's start by tossing aside whatever you've heard about low-fat, high-fat, or high-protein diets. For instance, the old diabetes recommendations included reducing the amount of fat you consume as a weight-loss strategy. However, replacing fat with more carbs actually causes diabetes to worsen and creates more body fat. That's why it is much more important to focus on controlling carbohydrates, which eventually turn into sugars that find their way into your blood and influence all your bodily functions.

Focusing your attention on carbohydrates doesn't mean that you don't need healthy proteins and fats, however. Every organ in your body has a preferred energy source derived from one of the three macronutrients. In fact, the right fats and proteins positively influence how your body functions throughout the day, as well as being integral to the carbohydrate story.

The major organs that consume, store, or affect blood glucose are the liver, brain, heart, fat tissues, muscles, and kidneys.

THE LIVER. This organ accounts for only 2 to 4 percent of your body weight, yet it is the most important organ in glucose regulation. It is where nutrients and other molecules absorbed from the gut are received and sorted. The liver absorbs nearly two-thirds of all glucose and almost all other carbohydrates that are absorbed in the intestine. It uses glucose to produce energy to power itself, and then converts excess glucose into glycogen. After the glycogen store is filled up, the liver converts more glucose into fatty acids or fat and makes antioxidants that promote better overall health. The liver can also make its own glucose from protein supplied from the muscles during the overnight fast and release it into the blood.

THE BRAIN. The brain needs a constant supply of glucose—around

100 to 120 grams every day—to function properly. But it can't store any glucose, which is why it has to constantly depend on the blood glucose for its energy needs. Not only that but also this blood glucose has to be kept above roughly 50 mg sugar/100mL of blood for it to be absorbed. If blood glucose levels fall below this number, brain cells cannot absorb glucose properly and can immediately starve and fail. This is why when we experience hypoglycemia, we feel dizzy, and we can pass out.

THE HEART. The heart actually prefers fat over glucose as fuel, but it still needs some glucose to function. Like the brain, it doesn't have much room for storage, so it has to constantly soak up glucose and fat from the blood. Yet too much fat, like too much glucose, in the blood can disrupt normal heart function.

BODY FAT. Fat tissues play an important role in glucose regulation. To successfully store fat in a nontoxic form, fat tissues need a little bit of glucose. The fat cells break glucose into smaller fragments and then use those small sugar bits to form three fatty-acid molecules known as triglycerides. Having an abundance of triglycerides can increase your risk for diabetes' sinister friend, heart disease. In another mechanism that occurs during the overnight fast, fat cells can release stored fat that travels to the liver to be used for energy production. A special type of fat tissue, called brown fat, is burned at night to warm the body.

MUSCLES. The muscles regulate glucose. Right after we eat, for the next 2 to 4 hours, the muscles soak up a large amount of glucose and store it as glycogen. When we use our muscles, particularly when we do moderate to intense exercise, it breaks down this glycogen for energy. When we are resting, though, our muscles prefer fat as an energy source. The more muscle you have and the more active you are, the more glucose you burn instead of storing it.

THE KIDNEYS. The kidneys filter the blood almost 60 times a day. During the process, the kidneys reabsorb glucose and necessary electrolytes from the blood. For these functions, the kidneys need a good amount of energy.

## WHAT YOU REALLY NEED TO KNOW ABOUT SUGAR

It would seem reasonable to say that if you are worried about diabetes, just eliminate carbs from your diet. Eating fewer carbs will certainly help lower your blood glucose, and that often accelerates weight loss.[1] However, we cannot completely stop eating carbohydrates, nor should we want to. Out of the three macronutrients, carbohydrates are most abundant in nature, and people typically consume nearly half of their daily calories as carbs. Yet too much sugar from carbohydrates causes swings in the blood glucose levels, so we get hungry more frequently and then cannot stick to an IF schedule; that is, we eat outside of our eating window. We've found that plenty of people can try to do IF, but in order to stay on IF and reap the benefits, they also have to refine their carb intake by eliminating the bad carbs from their diet. Just by making this one switch, you can bring your total carbohydrate intake down to a healthier level.

All plant foods contain carbohydrates. Whether you are eating spinach, rice, pasta, white potatoes, sweet potatoes, carrots, bananas, tomatoes, edamame (while you might have heard that soy is high in protein, 75 percent of edamame is carbs), peanuts, plums, cauliflower, bread, corn, honey, cane juice, or simple sugar, you are just eating carbs in different forms. When we eat plants, we not only get a lot of carbohydrates but we also get vitamins, minerals, antioxidants, fibers, protein, and fat—all the nutrients our body needs. For example, nuts are good sources of proteins and fat; and beans, berries, leafy green vegetables, quinoa, and whole grains are all good sources of fiber. Even rice, wheat, oats, and millet contain fiber, some protein, vitamins, and minerals.

The easiest carbs to digest are those that are quickly converted to glucose before the cells can use them to produce energy. Other carbs are very hard to digest or can never be fully digested. The carb that your body cannot easily digest is always the one to choose!

We can tell whether a carb is easy or hard to digest by the type of sugar it makes. Plants are packed with simple sugars created from sunlight, air, and water. All plants are made of cells that have a hard, impermeable cell wall that is mostly made of fiber. All the starches, or simple carbohydrates, that we get from plants are packed inside these cells; these are the ones which are easy to digest. The fibrous cell wall, which is considered a complex carbohydrate, is harder to digest. Complex carbohydrates need to be broken down into simple sugars, either by ripening, during digestion, or during industrial processing, in order to taste sweet.

When we eat fruits, vegetables, or nuts, it takes several steps to extract the nutrients from the carbs. In the first phase of chewing, we break down big pieces into smaller pieces of food particles and a little bit of simple sugar is released, which provides the sweet taste. The chewed food travels to the stomach, where it's broken down by the digestive juices for the next several minutes to hours. Once the cell walls break open, the nutrients stored inside the cells are released.

Different carbohydrates are broken down at different rates. The starches are the ones that easily convert to simple sugars; they are quickly absorbed in the gut and enter the bloodstream. The more complex carbohydrates that contain lots of fiber take more time to be broken down to simple sugars.

Complex carbs include raw fruits, vegetables, and nuts. Barley flours, millet flours, amaranth flour, whole wheat flour, rolled oats, and red or black rice have firmer seed coverings attached to them, and they are also considered complex carbohydrates. Wheat flour, rice flour, and corn flour have thin cell walls and little fiber, making them easier to digest. Cooking the plants also increases the amount of sugar that the body can easily obtain because the heat from cooking helps to break down the cell walls. For example, your stomach gets more carbohydrates and at a faster rate from eating cooked carrots or spinach as compared to eating raw carrots and spinach.

The fiber absorbs a lot of water and becomes a gooey mass that travels through the intestine and is essential for passing stool. During digestion, some of the fiber is broken down by trillions of microbes in the gut and used for their own food. The remaining passes in your stool. So, when you eat foods high in fiber, you are feeding the good bacteria in your gut and helping your body detoxify with regular bowel movements.

Other carbohydrate options, like grains, cannot be eaten until they are processed and pulverized, or *refined*, into a fine powder or flour. These flour molecules are so small that when we cook them, it is even easier for the stomach to quickly extract the sugar. What's more, during the refining process, these same flours lose the outer coating of the grains that had contained fiber, protein, fat and other nutrients. When cooked, these flours become very easy for the stomach to digest and quickly release sugar. The high-fiber grains that are slowly digested are the ones we will focus on to reverse diabetes, because the sugar from these grains enters the blood in a slower stream. For instance, when you eat whole grains like rolled or steel-cut oats, it's almost like switching on a drip system to water your plants. In contrast, a bowl of breakfast cereal is like choosing a fire hose to water those plants.

The negative impact of simple carbohydrates on diabetes is clear. We also know that eating lots of simple carbohydrates messes with the circadian rhythm. We have nicely documented the effect of simple carbohydrates in laboratory mice experiments. When mice are given a diet that is rich in complex carbohydrates and fiber along with other natural, whole foods, they typically eat fewer meals and eat less than 15 percent of their daily food intake during the day when they are supposed to sleep. When the same mice are given ultra-processed food containing 20 percent of their total calories from simple sugars, they eat smaller meals and eat them more frequently. In fact, they will eat 35 to 40 percent of their total food during the day when they are supposed to sleep. Even if we train the mice to eat within a particular window for weeks or months, as soon as they have access to food for 24 hours, the sugar in the diet brings back their old habit of eating around the clock.[2] It's the same with people, and that's why it is hard to stick with IF unless they make better food choices.

Carbs are present in almost everything we eat, and we cannot avoid consuming them when we are following a healthy diet packed with fruits and vegetables. The key is always going to be choosing the *right* carbs. If we eat foods that are packed with simple sugars or are ultra-processed, the sugar rush triggers the pancreas to release insulin, which can act on the circadian clock.[3] After the sugar and insulin rush dies down, the body swings into a low-sugar mode and feels hungry, so we eat again. Every time we eat, the insulin surge can nudge those clocks to run a little faster or slower. If these meals happen too many times over the course of a day, the clocks get confused and the bodily processes that should happen during the night or day get flipped—just as they did for the mice.

## FOODS TO AVOID

First, let's start with a quick overview of what you shouldn't be eating at all. These guidelines are true for everyone, especially for those with diabetes or a risk factor for developing it. Once those foods are out of the way, we can focus on all the great choices you and your family have for what to eat.

Take every item on this list that is currently sitting on your shelves and throw it away. If it's unopened, donate it to a food pantry near you. Sounds drastic? No, really, it's just six categories:

### 1. NO ULTRA-PROCESSED FOODS

One of the reasons why nearly 75 percent of U.S. adults are obese or overweight, and nearly half of U.S. adults are prediabetic (88 million) or have diabetes (34.2 million) is that we are living in a world where our most accessible food choices are bound to make us unhealthy. Ultra-processed foods are ready-to-eat foods that have been extracted from their original, natural form and then cooked in some fashion or combined with other ingredients, including some preservatives (to make them shelf stable). There are so many different types of ultra-processed foods that compiling a list of them seems futile. But we can use a simple rule of thumb when you are deciding which foods to avoid:

- The food does not resemble anything in nature.

- It comes in a package.

- You can eat it just by opening the package or by simply warming it/ microwaving it for a few minutes.

- It contains more than a handful of ingredients and you don't recognize the names of all of them.

An article in the *Wall Street Journal* claims that Americans eat as much as 58 percent of their calories from ultra-processed foods.[4] Yes, they are delicious. And eating them will not kill you ... right away. However, these foods will disrupt your circadian rhythm for when we should eat, and will lead to obesity and diabetes in four different ways:

1. Almost all contain highly addictive added ingredients, like sugar, so we tend to eat more of them. This includes "energy," protein, or any other variety of fruit and nut bars. They're just candy bars, even if they are marketed with pictures of triathletes or sports stars.

2. As we continue eating them, our total daily calorie intake goes up and exceeds the recommended daily intake. While we aren't counting calories, there is an upper limit for most of us of 2000 calories/ day before weight gain takes hold.

3. These foods are so processed that they are easily digested, leaving us hungry an hour or so after eating them, with the result that we eat more frequently at any time of the day or night. This eating pattern can disrupt sleep and the natural circadian rhythm, which further promotes cravings for these same unhealthy foods.

4. When you add points 1, 2, and 3, you are guaranteeing a rapid surge in blood glucose. This is why a bowl of oatmeal and a corn muffin may both be considered carbohydrates, but the oatmeal is much better for you and your blood glucose than a muffin.

## 2. NO SODA, DIET OR OTHERWISE

Drinking full-calorie sodas, sweetened ice teas, or sports drinks is one of the easiest and most effective methods to overconsume calories, main-line simple sugars into your body, and disrupt your blood glucose system. Other versions of these drinks with artificial sweeteners (see #6, opposite) are not healthier alternatives, as they are thought to change the good bacteria in your gut,[5] and your gut needs all the help it can get. If you feel like having a soda, try a sparkling water. Very refreshing!

## 3. NO PACKAGED FRUIT JUICES OR VEGETABLE JUICES

Even the ones that say they are "100 percent fruit juice" are not great choices, because most of these juices contain preservatives that can corrode your intestinal lining, causing leaky gut syndrome, and again messing with your gut's microbiome. Preservatives make food unpalatable for bacteria. But whatever is bad for bacteria outside your body may also be harmful to the bacteria inside your stomach, which can have other unwanted effects on your microbiome.

If you must have fruit or veggie juices, make them yourself and drink them the same day.

## 4. NO PRESWEETENED BREAKFAST CEREALS

I challenge you to find a commercial presweetened breakfast cereal that has fewer than 5 grams of sugar per serving. Most breakfast servings of ready-to-eat cereals have more than 10 percent sugar by weight.

## 5. NO ALCOHOL

All forms of alcohol affect the body's ability to process sugar. In fact, even drinks that aren't sweet, but are made from vegetables like potatoes (vodka) or plants (tequila), are still considered liquid sugars. When you drink beer, wine, or spirits, it disrupts the liver's process of sending glucose into the bloodstream. This may cause the blood sugar levels to fall, leading to hypoglycemia at some point over the next 12 hours. You know that feeling when you've drunk a little too much and you're off balance, dizzy, and your speech is affected? That's what hypoglycemia feels like.

And alcohol doesn't make a great pairing with some diabetes medications. If you have already been diagnosed with diabetes, alcohol can make the following complications worse:

- Damage to your kidneys
- Diabetic neuropathy
- Diabetic retinopathy
- High blood pressure
- High triglycerides

## 6. NO FOODS WITH ADDED SUGAR OR NON-SUGAR SWEETENERS

Read the nutrition labels on all the products in your pantry. Anything with added sugar is a no.

Sugars go by many names, but none of them are part of this program. Avoid foods made with:

| | |
|---|---|
| Agave syrup | Cane sugar or syrup |
| Aguamiel | Caramel or caramel color |
| All-natural sweetener | Clarified grape juice |
| Barbados molasses or sugar | Concentrated fruit juice |
| Beet sugar | Confectioner's sugar |
| Brown sugar | Cornstarch |

Corn sweetener

Corn syrup

Date sugar

Date syrup

Dextrin

Dextrose

Disaccharides

Evaporated cane juice

Fig syrup

Filtered honey

Fructose

Fruit juice concentrate

Fruit sugar

Fruit sweetener

Galactose

Glucose

Glycerin

Granulated sugar

Grape sugar

Guar gum

Heavy syrup

High fructose corn syrup

Hydrogenated glucose syrup

Inverted sugar or syrup

Jaggery

Lactose

Levulose

Light/lite sugar or syrup

Mannitol

Maple syrup

Modified food starch

Monosaccharides

Natural syrup

Nectars

Polysaccharides

Raisin syrup

Raw sugar

Ribbon cane syrup

Ribose

Rice malt

Rice syrup

Sorbitol

Sorghum molasses or syrup

Splenda

Sucrose

Turbinado sugar

Xylitol

There are a handful of artificial sugars that are okay to use in moderation to make some foods taste sweet. The downside of using them is that you may end up overeating these foods, because even artificial sweeteners can trigger food cravings. In this case, nothing is better than something, but if you have to have something, choose only from this list:

- Acesulfame-K (Ace-K, Sunett)

- Aspartame (Equal, NutraSweet)

- Monk fruit or Swingle fruit extract

- Neotame

- Saccharin (Sugar Twin, Sweet 'N Low)

- Sucralose (Splenda)

- Stevia (Truvia)

- Allulose/Swerve

### WHY SUPERMARKET WHOLE WHEAT BREAD MAY NOT ALWAYS BE A COMPLEX CARB

Switching your baking ingredients from all-purpose flour to whole wheat flour sounds like an improvement, but it's not a strategy to end diabetes. Neither is buying whole wheat bread from the supermarket. Whole wheat flour itself may be a complex carb, but when it's used in baking bread, for example, yeast is added for fermentation, which further breaks down the remaining complex starches into simple sugar. So, while you started with whole wheat, you end up with an ultra-processed food that creates the same sugar rush that you would have received from eating white bread.

If you are disappointed, you are not alone: one of my students participated in a recent study for which he was asked to wear a continuous glucose monitor. He was instructed to switch between white toast and whole wheat toast every day. He was thoroughly disappointed with his results: the whole wheat toast caused the same spikes in blood sugar as did the white toast.

## FOODS TO CHOOSE, AND WHEN TO EAT THEM

Now that you know what you can't eat, let's focus on what you can. An optimal IF day includes three meals that are well balanced and contain complex carbohydrates, lots of fiber, lean proteins, and healthy fats. That means during every meal, you need a bit of each of the macronutrients, although you'll see that some meals will lean more heavily on one or two. This is because different organs need various combinations of nutrients at distinct times of the day. It's all meant to support your circadian rhythm, as well as your blood sugar levels.

The backbone of this program is the popular Mediterranean diet. While there's no official, single diet that everyone living in the Mediterranean regions of Italy, Greece, Spain, Turkey, Morocco, and neighboring areas follows, the meal choices reflect a way of eating that people in this region have embraced over the centuries: combining fresh fruits and vegetables, beans and nuts, healthy grains, lean proteins, and dairy products. Simply choose the complex carbohydrates that are whole foods; proteins like eggs, fish, meat, and poultry; and monounsaturated fats that are liquid or soft at room temperature, like olive oil. The benefits of this plan are many: the diet is widely accepted as a heart-healthy eating plan,[6] and because you are eating only whole foods, it features the foods you need to eat in order to manage diabetes. And people who follow this type of dietary pattern are less likely to suffer from insomnia and shortened sleep,[7] so you will continue to make good food choices.

The general rule for this plan is very simple. By abiding by the 10- to 12-hour IF described in the previous chapter, you can have three meals and one snack every day. You will spread that allotment of calories in the following manner:

- A big breakfast: roughly 40 percent of all calories, eaten at least an hour after waking up

- A medium lunch: roughly 30 percent of all calories, eaten within the first half of your IF

- A medium dinner: roughly 25 percent of all calories, eaten at least 2 hours before you go to bed

- A small snack: roughly 5 percent of all calories, eaten in between any of these meals

You might be thinking, *Dr. Panda, you promised that I don't have to count calories. Now you are asking me to do so!* Well, not really. I don't want you to count calories, but you can guestimate by the size of the meals you are eating. It's not exactly scientific, but whatever your eating pattern is now, it's likely that you can increase your breakfast, decrease your lunch, and decrease your dinner. Keep reading to find out what you'll be eating in each of these meals. Remember, aligning your circadian code to optimize your body is always about the timing!

## KNOW BEFORE YOU GO (SHOPPING): THE GLYCEMIC INDEX

The glycemic index (GI) can be an IF follower's best friend. It is a rating system that standardizes how different carbohydrates affect blood sugar levels so that you can make better food choices. Most people cannot remember how they felt after eating one apple or one carrot, so the GI is a reference point to sort foods into categories to let you know if they are packed with simple sugars (high-GI foods) or if they contain complex carbohydrates (medium- or low-GI foods). High-GI carbohydrates result in spikes in blood sugar, causing a flood of insulin that triggers your body to store fat and become hungry again within several hours. In contrast, slow-burning, lower-GI foods cut your appetite and are more efficient at keeping glucose levels stabilized and insulin in check. Eating high-GI foods alone or even with healthier foods two to three times a day can bring a person close to prediabetes, accelerate the transition from prediabetes to diabetes, and worsen existing diabetes.[8] Avoiding high-GI foods and eating low-GI foods can lead to weight loss, especially in combination with IF.

The GI rating system isn't perfect, especially when it comes to packaged foods. The method for rating these foods is based on human trials. However, most of the tests were conducted on healthy young people who do not have diabetes. It is likely that some foods designated as medium/moderate GI may not be good for people concerned about diabetes. This is why all the foods I recommend, and that are listed on the Shopping List (see page 142) are considered low-, or ultra-low-GI foods.

## PLAY THE LOW-GLYCEMIC GAME

You can find a full GI index at GlycemicIndex.com/GI-Search. It's useful for determining how to swap out the foods you can't eat and choose their healthier versions. For instance, in my family, we have switched from traditional basmati rice, which is highly processed and has a high GI, to parboiled rice. The latter is considered a complex carbohydrate because it is difficult to digest. It has the same healthy components as brown rice, which is another good alternative to white rice.

I know that giving up your favorite foods is difficult. In fact, many people in our studies report that it's harder to eat low-glycemic foods than to follow IF. One strategy is to start your IF 12-week program without changing your food choices. Then, in Week 3, start to slowly adopt more low-glycemic choices. By Week 4, you may find that you have eliminated all medium- and high-glycemic foods on your own, because you are already seeing how much better you feel.

## ANITA AND NEEL EASILY SWAPPED LOW-QUALITY CARBS FOR COMPLEX CARBS

Anita and her husband Neel are engineers at a California tech company. They are in their mid-30s and lead very busy lives. They both wanted to have a baby, so they decided to have their annual physicals before they tried to conceive. Their test results were shocking and unexpected: they were both prediabetic. This was a problem because for both men and women, being diabetic makes it more difficult to conceive.

Their typical lifestyle was to start the day with a cup of tea with cream and sugar and a cookie right after getting out of bed. Then they would rush to work, where their company provided lots of free food any time of the day or night, so they ate most of their meals in the office. Their favorite foods were granola or cereal with milk, fruit juices, coffee, protein bars, pizza, club sandwiches, trail mixes, and anything else that could be eaten while they sat next to their computer keyboards. In the evening they would order takeout from an Indian restaurant: they had basmati rice and some type of curry. After finishing dinner around 8 p.m., they would go back to work on their laptops and later get to relax and watch some TV with ice cream or some sweet treats before bedtime.

Neel suggested that they immediately start a 10-hour IF to reverse their diagnoses. They had heard that some people can do IF without changing their diet, so they liked that idea. However, they struggled to adopt IF with their usual diet. Even though they skipped their morning tea and delayed their breakfast till 10:00 a.m., and had their favorite basmati rice and curry dishes by 8:00 p.m., they had their hunger pangs at 10:00 p.m., and could not stop eating the after-dinner snacks and sweets until they went to bed around midnight.

Worse, when they went back to the doctor a couple of months later, their blood glucose levels did not budge. That's when Anita reached out to me. She had heard me speak on a podcast. She wanted some tips about adopting IF with their usual food, but I told her they weren't going to get great results if they continued to follow this kind of high-glycemic, high-carb diet. They didn't realize that their sugary snacks, fruit juices, and basmati rice were causing big swings in their blood sugar levels, which was making it difficult for them to resist their late-night hunger pangs. I explained that the best way to stay on a strict IF was to swap out at least some of these foods, and I made a couple of suggestions. I told them about my favorite overnight oats and cottage cheese for breakfast, nuts for snacks, and salad with walnuts or lentil burgers for lunch; further, I suggested substituting whole wheat Indian bread (roti) for the basmati rice.

A couple of weeks later I received another text from Anita. By following my suggestions, they found that their new diet made a huge difference. Now that they were getting plenty of complex carbs and fewer simple ones, it became easier for them to successfully adopt a 10-hour IF, as they no longer got late-night hunger pangs. They also realized that many low-glycemic food choices were available right at work, once they were able to look past the pizza and sandwich stations.

Anita and Neel have kept in touch with me. They now have a baby girl and are expecting another baby. They've stayed on their IF with better food choices, and now they are both diabetes-free.

## WHAT TO EAT: BREAKFAST

When you start intermittent fasting, you may want to eat a big breakfast because you're hungry from the overnight fast. This is not a problem, and in fact, I encourage it. On this plan you will be having the majority of your calories in the first half of your eating window. Here's an example: if your 10-hour IF is going to be from 8:00 a.m. to 6:00 p.m., then you aim to finish lunch by 1:00 p.m. (5 hours into your IF) and then you've had most of your calories in the first half of the eating window.

There is a circadian reason for this: in the first half of the day, the pancreas produces more insulin and at night it slows down. IF aligns the pancreas clock to be more sensitive to food and produce more insulin in the first half of the eating window. In one recent study, researchers found that when people shift to eating most of the macronutrients in the early hours of the day, they saw improved blood work and reduced body weight, along with a reduction in overall appetite and better glucose control for those with Type 2 diabetes.[9] Eating a big breakfast aligns with the pancreas clock, and the blood insulin level does not rise too high. After you eat a big breakfast, you have the whole day to get some activity and exercise, so your muscles will help you to absorb those extra calories.

And because your insulin response is better in the morning, and nearly half the food you will eat all day is carbohydrates, you are taking advantage of that insulin response when your body can process carbs better by eating a breakfast that includes lots of complex carbs. In the same study, we found that an increased complex carbohydrate intake at breakfast and a reduced complex carbohydrate intake at dinner improved overall blood glucose control and weight loss, and also reduced hunger and cravings, compared with a reverse schedule.

Remember, not any carb will do. Choose only from the low- and ultra-low-GI carbs, like fiber-rich oatmeal made from old-fashioned rolled or steel-cut oats, to help control blood sugar throughout the day. Vegetables, fruits, nuts, and seeds easily add more complex carbs to your plate. Combine these great carb choices with protein, as well. Eating protein early in the day triggers the right amount of acid secretion in the stomach. If you have more protein at breakfast than at dinner, you will reduce your chance of getting heartburn or a poor night's sleep. This combination actually makes your digestive system work longer to digest food, and you will feel full (satiated and less hungry) for hours and will be less likely to snack.

My go-to breakfast is a combination of oatmeal, cottage cheese, and almond powder (that I make myself by crushing almonds in a coffee grinder). This works for me because the cottage cheese has a lot of protein, and the oatmeal and almond powder are both low glycemic. When I want an extra carb hit, I throw in a handful of blueberries.

Other great breakfast choices are:

- Cottage cheese with fruit

- Hard-boiled eggs and fruit

- Low-glycemic toast, like Ezekiel brand breads, with cheese, avocado, or peanut butter

- Prepared oatmeal with nuts/seeds

- Unflavored/unsweetened yogurt (any type) with fruit/nuts/seeds

- Vegetable omelet

## WHAT TO EAT: LUNCH

Your next meal needs to get you through the rest of the day without your having to snack and can support an afternoon workout. You also want to avoid the after-lunch low if your work is primarily sedentary. We've found that a lunch that is smaller than breakfast and is high in protein and lower in carbs and fat (but that includes some) is the best way to go.

For example, enjoy all different types of high-quality protein sources with complex carb vegetables. Think about a salad with your favorite protein or a stir-fry. The foods highest in protein include animal meats, poultry, fish, seafood, beans and peas, eggs, soy, nuts, and seeds. Leafy green vegetables and dairy also contain protein. Animal proteins are the richest source of protein, though.

Is it possible to eat too much protein? Yes. The rule of thumb for daily intake is 0.36 gram of protein per day per pound of body weight. So, for someone who weighs around 150 pounds, that would be about 56 grams of protein a day. Most of us are eating at least that amount of protein.[10] For example, one large cooked egg has 6 grams of protein and a cooked quarter-pound hamburger patty has roughly 16 grams of protein.

Eating too much protein is hard on your kidneys, and you really would like to go through life with two working kidneys. When protein is used in the body, its by-products, including urea, are not needed, so such waste products are filtered out into urine by the kidneys. So, too much protein intake with weak kidneys can cause waste to build up in the blood. In some diabetic patients, weak kidneys may not be able to remove all the extra waste. Therefore, it is important to eat just the right amount of protein each day to nourish your body, without putting extra stress on your kidneys. As mentioned, the amount of protein you need is based on your body size, the health of your kidneys, and the amount of protein that may be in your urine. Ask your dietitian or health-care provider to tell you exactly how much protein you should eat every day.

However, there are two particular groups of people who may need to consume slightly more protein during lunch. If you are already diabetic and 50 years or older, eating more protein can help increase muscle mass. This group of people need 1 gram per kilogram of body weight—a much higher amount of protein—to support physical activity that builds and retains muscle mass.[11] However, you still need to consider the source. Protein drinks sound like a good idea to maintain muscle mass. However, they can also contain a lot of ingredients you don't really want. One popular shake mix has 15 grams of protein and 10 grams of sugar. If you feel you need a protein drink, choose one that doesn't contain added sugar or sugar substitutes.

Vegetarians need to pay special attention to ensuring they are eating enough protein. The vegetarian choices with the greatest amount of protein include tofu, cottage cheese, and lentils. However, lentils are only 25 percent protein and almost 65 percent complex carbohydrates. So, while they're a healthy choice and will keep you feeling full, you have to eat a lot in order for them to count as a "high-protein" choice.

Some great lunch choices include:

- Bean and vegetable stew
- Burrito bowl (skip the rice) with beans, fajita vegetables, chicken or tofu, lettuce, avocado, and salsa
- Green salad with tomatoes, cucumber, red onion, feta cheese, and grilled fish
- Kale salad with grilled chicken breast
- Moussaka (eggplant casserole with a béchamel sauce)
- Stir-fried tofu and brown rice

---

**COMBINE INTERMITTENT FASTING WITH A KETO DIET**

When the body runs out of readily available or stored carbohydrates, the liver can break down both dietary fat and body fat to produce smaller fat molecules called ketones. Ketones are a good source of energy and they can be used efficiently by many organs and, to some extent, by the brain. Typically, the ketone level in the blood is relatively low (<0.6 millimole/L), but when you are following a 10-hour IF, your liver produces a modest number of ketones (blood ketone 0.6–1.5 millimole/L). IF itself will bring your body to a ketogenic state that lasts for a few hours toward the end of your overnight fast, allowing you to burn fat and lose weight.

This same modest number of ketones in the blood sends a signal to the rest of the body that we have run out of stored glucose, and it gears up for survival mode. As a result, the immune system gets a boost and the nerve cells produce hormone-like molecules called brain-derived neurotropic factor (BDNF) to strengthen the nerve cells and their connections. This improves cognitive function; we can think clearly and get a good night's sleep.

You can boost ketone production beyond what you can get with IF and a standard diet (between 1.5 and 3.0 millimole/L) by eating a very-low carbohydrate ketogenic diet, which is a significant jump from the eating plan in this book. A very-low-carb keto diet is less than 20 grams of carbs a day, and most of the calories are from fat and protein. To do this means you have to get rid of almost all grains and eat only fruits and vegetables that are rich in fiber.

If you are on diabetes medications, consult with your doctor before you start a ketogenic diet, because you may need to adjust your medications and then check in with the doctor regularly. And if you cannot continue on a ketogenic diet, don't worry. Sticking with IF is an effective lifelong strategy.

## WHAT TO EAT: DINNER

One of the biggest questions we get about IF is whether people are hungry before bed or during the overnight fast, especially if the fast starts early in the evening. This is of concern if you are also trying to decrease the size of your dinner. The changes to what you are eating for dinner, and when you are eating, are probably the biggest disruptions to a standard eating routine. You can expect that during the first week of IF you might feel hungry later in the evening before you go to bed. Almost all of our study participants have said that the first week is the hardest to get through. But afterward, your body will adapt to better circadian alignment and you will not feel hungry anymore.

One way we address this issue of late-night hunger is by creating a dinner meal that is higher in protein and fat, and that includes fewer carbohydrates (but not none!). This combination will help you get through the evening and overnight fast without feeling hungry. Dietary fats are the macronutrients that keep you feeling full and satisfied. What's more, mixing healthy fats with vegetables can make both more palatable and satisfying. You can also puree steamed vegetables in a blender or food processor, add some cheese and butter, or flavored olive oil, and create a hearty soup.

Having a dinner that includes fats is not an invitation to have ice cream every night. Ice cream is an ultra-processed food that is loaded with simple sugars or sugar substitutes. Nor is dark chocolate/hot chocolate in the evening a good idea. One 5-ounce bar of dark chocolate has the same amount of caffeine as in a cup of coffee. If you love your chocolate, have milk chocolate, which has half the caffeine as dark chocolate.

Some great dinner choices include:

- Brown rice with lentils (dal) and sautéed vegetables
- Clam chowder
- Grilled vegetables and paneer (Indian pressed cottage cheese)
- Meat and bean enchilada made with a whole wheat tortilla
- Sausage, winter squash, and spinach
- Whole wheat spaghetti with homemade meatballs and tomato sauce (make sure the meatballs and tomato sauce don't contain corn syrup or added sugar)

## WHAT TO EAT: SNACKS

If you must snack in between meals, try any of these low-glycemic options. One of my favorite tricks is to eat nuts that come in shells. The effort it takes to break open the shells takes time and you end up eating fewer nuts.

Some other great options are:

- Cup of lentil soup or vegetable broth
- Hard-boiled eggs
- Low-glycemic bread or crackers with hummus
- Low-glycemic bread with cheese
- Peanuts
- Pistachio nuts
- Plain whole-milk yogurt or Greek yogurt
- Whole fruits (orange, apple, pear, peach, etc.)

## DRINK LOTS OF WATER WITH EVERY MEAL

Your body needs a lot of water throughout the day, and hydration has a circadian component. We are more likely to feel thirsty during the day because the body needs water to digest and process nutrients. It's a good idea to have a glass of water every hour or two so that you stay hydrated and energetic, especially through the afternoon, when you might be exercising. If you find water too bland, you can have herbal teas throughout the day, iced or hot. You can also add a squeeze of lemon or lime, or a bit of 100% fruit juice to make it more palatable. The goal is to have eight 8-ounce glasses of water a day.

Drinking water after dinner doesn't disrupt your eating window, and it will not make you wake up in the middle of the night, either. And if you wake up in the middle of the night and feel thirsty, go ahead and drink some water. I've found that if I wake up thirsty but I don't drink water, then I will stay awake. If I drink water, it's likely I will go back to sleep right away.

I don't count coffee as a water source, as coffee itself can make us feel dehydrated and suppress sleep. Decaffeinated herbal teas may count toward water intake, however. Some people like a cup of herbal tea before bed, and as long as it doesn't have any caffeine, sweeteners, or milk, it's an acceptable option. Regular tea actually has a good amount of caffeine—the same ingredient in coffee that keeps us awake—and even some herbal teas have caffeine. Read labels carefully and make choices that support your code.

## THE CIRCADIAN DIABETES CODE SHOPPING LIST

Many people who are diabetic, want to prevent diabetes, or want to lose weight often say that "healthy food" tastes bad. The first image of healthy food in their mind is typically all the things they don't like to eat. Many people have told me they don't want to give up french fries and ketchup for carrots and broccoli. But when I tell them all the wonderful foods other than carrots and broccoli that they can eat, they always find something they enjoy. So, look at the list carefully and check the foods you already like. Then try one or two new options each week so as to round out your diet.

Everything on this list is considered to be low glycemic. Nothing on this list is hard to find or unavailable in any supermarket. You'll see that there are plenty of healthy choices and you will always find something healthy to eat that's within your eating window, putting you in control of your blood sugar.

## GRAINS AND GRAIN PRODUCTS

| | |
|---|---|
| Brown rice | Rice (converted, parboiled) |
| Bulgur | Rye |
| Ezekiel bread | Rye Bread |
| Multigrain bread | Sourdough bread |
| Mung bean noodles | Spelt bread |
| Oats (steel-cut or old-fashioned rolled oats have the highest amount of fiber) | Whole grain/ whole wheat/ corn tortillas |
| | Whole wheat pasta |
| Pearled barley | Wild rice |
| Popcorn | |

## FRUITS AND VEGETABLES

| | |
|---|---|
| Apples | Artichokes |
| Apricots | Arugula |

| | |
|---|---|
| Asparagus | Mangoes |
| Avocados | Mushrooms |
| Beet greens | Mustard greens |
| Blackberries | Okra |
| Blueberries | Olives |
| Bok choy | Onions |
| Broccoli | Oranges |
| Brussels sprouts | Peaches |
| Cabbage | Pears |
| Cantaloupe | Peppers (all varieties) |
| Cauliflower | Plums |
| Celery | Pomegranates |
| Collard greens | Prunes |
| Cucumbers | Radishes |
| Eggplant | Raspberries |
| Fennel | Romaine lettuce |
| Fiddleheads | Rutabaga |
| Garlic | Sea vegetables (dulse, kelp) |
| Grapefruit | Spinach |
| Honeydew melon | Strawberries |
| Jerusalem artichokes | Summer squash |
| Jicama | Sweet potatoes |
| Kale | Swiss chard |
| Leeks | Tangerines |

Tomatoes

Turnips and turnip greens

Watercress

Winter squash

Zucchini

## VEGETARIAN OPTIONS HIGH IN PROTEIN

Black beans

Black-eyed peas

Butter beans

Garbanzo beans (chickpeas)

Green beans

Kidney beans

Lentils

Lima beans

Mung beans

Navy beans

Peanuts

Pinto beans

Romano beans

Snow peas

Soy (tofu, edamame, and dried soybeans)

Split peas

Sugar snap peas

White beans

Also, pastas made from beans (black bean, chickpea, lentil, etc.)

## PROTEIN FROM ANIMAL SOURCES

Beef

Bison/buffalo

Chicken

Duck

Eggs

Lamb

Pork

Turkey

Veal

## PROTEIN FROM FISH AND SHELLFISH

| | |
|---|---|
| Catfish | Octopus |
| Clams | Oysters |
| Cod | Pollock |
| Crab | Salmon |
| Crayfish | Scallops |
| Flounder | Sea bass |
| Haddock | Shrimp |
| Halibut | Snapper |
| Herring | Squid (calamari) |
| Lobster | Swordfish |
| Mackerel | Trout |
| Mussels | Tuna |

## DAIRY PRODUCTS

| | |
|---|---|
| Almond milk (unsweetened) | Milk (whole) |
| Butter | Oat milk (unsweetened) |
| Buttermilk | Plain yogurt (any style) |
| Cottage cheese (unflavored) | Sour cream |
| Cheese | Soy milk |

## NUTS, NUT BUTTERS, AND SEEDS

| | |
|---|---|
| Almonds | Peanuts |
| Brazil nuts | Pecans |
| Chestnuts | Pine nuts |
| Chia seeds | Pistachios |
| Flax seeds | Pumpkin seeds |
| Hazelnuts | Sesame seeds |
| Hemp seeds | Sunflower seeds |
| Nut butters | Walnuts |

## HEALTHY FATS AND OILS

| | |
|---|---|
| Avocado oil | Macadamia oil |
| Butter | Olive oil |

## TIPS FOR EATING OUTSIDE YOUR HOME

The challenge with eating out is that most restaurants—from fast-food joints to high-end eating establishments—serve food that is loaded with ultra-processed ingredients and contains too many calories. A recent survey by the National Heart, Lung, and Blood Institute (NHLBI) found that many popular foods and restaurant meals have nearly doubled in calorie content over the last three decades.

. If you are planning on eating out or bringing prepared foods home, always look for a place that has hearty salads and vegetables, tofu, fish, or lean meat options on the menu. You can also trim the calories by ordering one entrée to share with someone or take half home to eat at another time. Lastly, you don't have to order a three-course meal. With most portions being supersized, you can comfortably choose a main course or pick one or two items from the first-course offerings. If you must have the dessert, berries or a cheese plate are good options.

Another challenge comes up when you are invited to someone else's home. Many of us were taught that it is impolite to refuse food that is offered. But if you are a vegetarian and someone offers you a hot dog, you can decline and the host will understand. Similarly, when offered foods at times that are outside your IF window or would be a high-glycemic meal, you can simply say that you have finished eating for the day, and instead enjoy some herbal tea or sparkling water while others eat and drink. Eating and drinking are part of the social fabric of life, and you have to make the best choices for you. There's no need to feel embarrassed about doing IF; feel free to tell everyone you know that you are taking care of your health, and that it's making you feel much better. They'll understand and be happy for you!

During social events when you cannot choose when you eat, you can still choose what to eat. Make the healthiest choices from what's available, and stay away from alcohol, sugary drinks, cake, and ultra-processed foods. Hold a glass of water, sparkling water, or herbal tea with pride. If going to parties is too stressful, host your own! Instead of offering dinner, invite people for brunch, lunch, or an early dinner. Then, you can control both the when and the what you eat.

## WHAT'S NEXT

Now you are up to date on the latest wisdom about food and diabetes. In the next chapter, we'll combine IF with exercise for achieving even better health.

## CHAPTER 7

# When to Exercise

Exercise can be as powerful as intermittent fasting (IF) when it comes to reversing diabetes and its complications. In fact, molecular analyses of what happens to the organs and blood glucose levels show that IF and exercise have many similar benefits.[1] Both help to reduce blood glucose, improve heart function, nurture the liver, boost the immune system, and support brain health. When you combine IF with exercise, the benefits to your diabetes and related health conditions are exponential: exercise boosts the benefits of IF, and IF boosts the benefits of exercise.

Exercise also improves muscle mass, muscle strength, bone health, motor coordination, metabolism, gut function, heart health, and lung capacity. Exercise literally relaxes the brain, reducing depression and anxiety and increasing your ability to experience happiness. What's more, exercise has a circadian effect, improving sleep and mood. In this chapter, you'll learn when to exercise and how to support your activity.

## EXERCISE IMPROVES DIABETES

According to the American Diabetes Association (ADA), regular exercise may prevent or delay Type 2 diabetes development.[2] It improves blood glucose control, reduces cardiovascular risk factors, contributes to weight loss, and improves the well-being of people with Type 2 diabetes.[3,4] Regular exercise also has considerable health benefits for people with Type 1 diabetes, including improved cardiovascular fitness, muscle strength, and insulin sensitivity.[5]

Exercise improves blood glucose levels by way of many different mechanisms. First, during exercise and for the next 30 to 60 minutes, your muscles absorb glucose with very little help from insulin. This means that most diabetics who have enough insulin, but whose organs are not sensitive to insulin, will benefit from exercise, as it opens a backdoor to allow glucose to enter the muscles without help from insulin. Those who make less insulin also benefit, because they may need fewer medications to pump out insulin from their pancreas. Finally, Type 1 diabetics or insulin-dependent diabetics may find that they need fewer insulin injections to control their blood glucose. So, exercise can reduce your reliance on medication or insulin to control diabetes. However, you have to keep up the exercise habit, because the benefits build daily and you can lose them if you go back to your previous sedentary life.

Exercise increases the capillary bed in the muscles so that glucose becomes available for cells to use.[6] Better blood circulation to the muscles also brings nutrients and hormones to support muscle repair and muscle growth, which is what happens as you add more strength exercises to your routine. Since the muscles are the largest organ that absorbs glucose, having more muscle helps to control blood glucose and reduce diabetes.

## STARTING AN EXERCISE PROGRAM IS OFTEN THE HARDEST PART

Just like the organs need a healthy level of blood glucose to operate efficiently, the joints need a healthy level of blood glucose. So, when blood glucose levels increase, as happens in diabetes, the joints are one of the first parts of the body to suffer that is easily noticed. Muscles are connected to bones by tendons, and the bones are connected to each other with ligaments. The ligaments and tendons are made of long strands of collagen fiber, and they need a healthy level of blood glucose to function normally. When blood glucose levels increase, the glucose can stick to the collagen fibers,[7] just like an iron wire gets coated with rust over time.

When this sticky glucose builds up for months or years, your joints will feel stiff, or you may have pain in your hips, knees, heels, elbows, shoulders, fingers, or wrists. Any pain or stiffness in these locations will make exercise unenjoyable, if not difficult.

What's more, each time you exercise, you create a tiny bit of damage to your muscles and joints, then those muscles and joints repair themselves with the help of your immune cells that clean up the mess. But as you learned in Chapter 1, diabetes also affects the body's immune response, making it hyperactive and causing additional inflammation, particularly to these same joints. This is another reason why it is so critical to take your health seriously: while others may dismiss joint pain as an outcome of getting older, it's not a normal body function. In fact, it is likely that high blood glucose is causing it.

If you have joint pain that makes exercise challenging right now, don't worry. After four or five weeks of IF, your blood glucose may reduce and your immune cells will be less inflammatory. You will feel less joint pain, which will make moving and exercising easier. You may also find that afternoon exercise is more comfortable than morning exercise, as the body is warmer in the afternoon, the joints are more flexible, and you'll experience less joint pain.

Starting an exercise program is often the hardest part, but as you'll see, the benefits are enormous. Once you begin and you start seeing the results of your efforts on both your diabetes and your circadian code, you will be over the initial hurdle and well on your way to creating a new, sustainable habit.

## EXERCISE ENHANCES SLEEP AND CIRCADIAN RHYTHMS

Anyone who does a lot of physical activity during the day knows that the activity makes it relatively easy to fall asleep at night. Even sedentary people who spend a full day in an amusement park report a better night's sleep. A few years back, circadian scientists wanted to find out what actually caused this relationship. Some of the earliest experiments examining the effect of physical activity on circadian rhythm and sleep were done on mice that had free access to an exercise wheel. When these mice hopped on the exercise wheel whenever they wanted, they voluntarily ran on the wheel every night (remember, mice are nocturnal). Researchers found that the exercising mice had a robust circadian clock; they slept better during the day when they are supposed to and were less sleepy when they were meant to stay awake.[8] The effect of physical activity on sleep did not seem to involve food and it didn't affect their thirst.

This early observation prompted several human studies involving a range of participants, from teenagers to older adults. All the studies have led to the same conclusion: physical activity improves sleep. Among teenagers, vigorous physical activity not only improved how quickly they fell asleep or how well they slept but it also improved their mood during the day, increased their ability to concentrate, and reduced their levels of anxiety and depressive symptoms.[9] Among older adults (50 to 75 years old), moderate physical activity or even regular stretching improved sleep onset, sleep quality, and sleep duration, and also reduced dependence on sleep medications. Older adults with moderate physical activity also had fewer episodes of feeling sleepy during regular daytime activity.[10,11,12]

Those with sleep disorders might find that exercise has a strong influence on their circadian code. Even those just starting a new exercise program may find that they go to sleep more quickly and wake up less often at night. For instance, studies show that after exercise, the cells inside the muscles produce several molecules, including interleukin-15 (IL-15), which increases bone mass. Interestingly, IL-15 also has some benefits for sleep. In one study, rabbits injected with a small amount of IL-15 were found to have better and deeper sleep.[13]

A second mechanism that promotes better sleep occurs when the muscle cells produce another molecule, irisin. People with diabetes often have less muscle mass and produce less irisin. Reduced amounts of irisin correlate with obstructive sleep apnea.[14] However, when people build more muscle mass, they can also reduce sleep apnea, which promotes a better night's sleep.[15]

Another mechanism by which exercise improves sleep may be through the liver and the hormone-like molecule BDNF. Prolonged exercise can trigger the production of healthy levels of ketone bodies in the liver, which tells the brain to produce BDNF.[16] A higher level of BDNF makes the connections between the brain cells stronger and also promotes better sleep.

New research is showing that *when* you choose to exercise can positively impact sleep. When we exercise, our body temperature goes up; after exercise, our core body temperature drops. The body needs to cool down in order for us to fall asleep. Therefore, late afternoon/early evening exercise provides plenty of time to cool down before bed, which may help to improve nightly sleep.[17]

If you have insomnia, see your doctor before you begin a new physical activity program. Insomnia increases the risk of heart disease and stroke, and an exercise program should be done under a doctor's supervision.

## THE CIRCADIAN COMPONENT FOR MAINTAINING STRENGTH

An enhanced circadian rhythm helps maintain strength so that we are physically fit enough to exercise. The body's physical strength is largely determined by the overall mass and health of the cartilage, bones, and muscles, each of which has its own circadian clock that sets a rhythm for repair and rebuilding. For example, cartilage cells don't have the luxury of multiplying as often as other cells in the body (such as blood cells, liver cells, etc.). These cells produce the gluelike material that forms the cushion between bones. As we move around, this cushion experiences regular wear and tear. The cartilage cells make this glue on a daily rhythm, with more produced during the night. When the circadian clock is disrupted, this repair process is diminished,[18] which can lead to osteoarthritis.

Bones also go through a daily repair process, which is different from cartilage repair. Bones are made of minerals, including calcium, that are secreted by its cells. Another type of bone cell eats up damaged bone. The circadian clocks in the bone cells are synchronized so that bone making and bone eating do not occur at the same time of the day. What's more, the balance between these two cell types is important: too much bone eating can lead to bone loss, while too much bone making can push against the other bones and create additional damage near the joints. When the circadian clock is disrupted, the bone-making cells are not fully activated, and they don't produce enough raw materials for making new bone. Similarly, the bone-eating cells are not fully activated, so they don't clear all the damaged bone material completely. This ultimately leads to weaker bones that are prone to fracture.

The circadian clock also plays a crucial role in both the formation of new muscle fiber and in muscle function. Clock genes directly regulate other genes that are necessary for making new muscle cells or muscle fibers. Clock genes also determine the type of muscles we have. That is, we typically have two types of muscles: slow-twitch (type I) muscles are rich in mitochondria and help us perform endurance exercise or marathon running; fast-twitch (type II) muscles contain less mitochondria but help us when we are sprinting. Having a better clock appears to increase the function of slow-twitch muscles.[19]

A healthy circadian clock nurtures the muscles both after eating and during the overnight fast. After a meal, the muscle clock activates the function of the metabolic genes involved in the absorption and utilization of glucose and dietary fat, which fuels muscle function.[20] During the overnight fast, the circadian clock instructs other genes to break down damaged muscle proteins and send them to the liver for recycling while we are sleeping. The clock also helps produce new muscle proteins and ensures that the fibers are properly aligned for coherent movement. With all these important roles for the circadian clock in muscle structure and function, it is not surprising that mice lacking a functional clock in their muscles cannot exercise enough and get tired too soon.[21] In people, we know that poor sleep and circadian disruption negatively impact exercise performance.[22]

Just like the circadian clock nurtures the muscle and bones, new research shows it also nurtures the joints by repairing damage to tendons and ligaments. These connective tissues are maintained by secretion of collagens, their organization into long fibers that support the joints, and degradation of damaged collagens at different times of the day. Having a healthy circadian code supports these collagens, which in turn supports flexible and strong joints.[23]

On the other hand, exercise can increase the level of an enzyme involved in the production of heme, the pigment in the blood that carries oxygen to all the tissues.[24] The same pigment is also an important part of the circadian code, as it delivers the signal to turn on and off different genes involved in the metabolism of glucose and fat, as well as the production of hormonelike molecules from muscles that can go through the bloodstream to affect function of other organs or the brain. This is one of the ways exercise can enhance the muscle clock.

## TYPES OF EXERCISE THAT REVERSE OR MANAGE DIABETES

Exercise doesn't have to be rigorous or complicated. The ADA believes, as I do, that physical activity can be anything that makes you move your body and burn calories. This includes a vast range of activities, from climbing stairs to playing organized sports.

There are three basic types of physical activity:

AEROBIC EXERCISE. Rhythmic in nature, aerobic exercise includes anything that gets your heart rate up for a sustained period of time. Regular, moderate aerobic activity like walking, cycling, jogging, or swimming is associated with substantially lower cardiovascular risks in both Type 1 and Type 2 diabetes. In Type 1 diabetes, aerobic training increases cardiorespiratory fitness, decreases insulin resistance, and improves heart function.[25] For those with Type 2 diabetes, aerobic training improves heart health, lowers blood pressure, and improves insulin resistance.[26] High-intensity interval training (HIIT), which is a method of performing more intense aerobic activity over very short periods of time (like a minute or two with rests in between) is also thought to further improve insulin sensitivity and glycemic control in adults with both Type 1 and Type 2 diabetes.[27,28] Since exercise helps the muscles soak up blood glucose with very little help from insulin, short bouts of aerobic exercise after every meal can be as effective as many diabetes medicines. These short bouts can be as brief as 10 minutes of walking around the block or getting on a treadmill or an elliptical.

STRENGTH OR RESISTANCE TRAINING. This type of exercise increases muscle mass and overall stamina. It consists of short, high-intensity activity and relies on energy sources that are stored in the muscles. Diabetes influences your muscle mass and muscle strength. When the body has to break down muscle protein for the liver to make additional glucose, your muscle mass and muscle strength may decrease. Therefore, everyone with diabetes should do some daily strength exercise to maintain or build muscle mass and strengthen their muscles. Those without diabetes will also benefit because increasing muscle mass can reduce the risk for developing diabetes.

STRETCHING, FLEXIBILITY, AND BALANCE. These types of exercises improve joint mobility and allow you to increase participation in strength-training exercises. Standardized stretching practices yield the best results. For instance, yoga is thought to promote improvement in glycemic control for people with Type 2 diabetes.[29] Tai chi may improve glycemic control and neuropathic symptoms for those with Type 1 diabetes, as well as those with neuropathy.[30]

Unless you recently have had a heart attack or stroke or been diagnosed with severe heart disease, the ADA says that all adults need *at least* 150 minutes per week of moderate exercise, or 75 minutes per week of vigorous exercise (or a combination of both). That breaks down to moderate exercise for 30 minutes a day, five times a week, or more. This recommendation only takes into account the aerobic exercise piece of the equation.

Based on research, I believe the optimal diabetes exercise program must include some movement every day. The chart that follows, adapted from the 2016 ADA recommendations, illustrates the best way to combine aerobic exercise, strength training, and flexibility. Consider this the minimum recommendation: it never hurts and always helps to move more.

## YOUR CIRCADIAN CODE WEEKLY EXERCISE ROUTINE

|  | Aerobic Exercise | Resistance/Strength Training | Stretching, Flexibility, and Balance |
|---|---|---|---|
| Suggested Exercises | Walking<br>Cycling<br>Swimming<br>Jogging<br>Racquet sports<br>Zumba/Dance | Resistance machines<br>Free weights<br>Resistance bands<br>Body weight as resistance exercises | Yoga<br>Tai Chi |
| Intensity | Moderate to vigorous<br>May be done continuously or as HIIT | Moderate: 15 repetitions of an exercise that can be repeated no more than 15 times<br>Vigorous: 8 repetitions of an exercise that can be repeated no more than 8 times | Light to moderate intensity |
| Duration and Frequency | At least 150 mins./week<br>Can be broken into segments of at least 3 days a week | At least 3 days a week, with a day off in between each day<br>8 different exercises, 1 to 3 sets of 8 repetitions | 1 day a week of 1-hour guided exercise |

## TAKE A WALK

The simplest exercise is walking, and almost everyone can add more walking to their daily routine. Unless you have heart issues or vertigo, you don't need a doctor's permission to take a walk. Try to keep up a brisk pace, whereby it would be difficult to carry on a conversation while walking. Thirty minutes of brisk walking should be 4,500 to 5,000 steps, which is a reasonable goal. When it comes to exercise, more is always better.

All kinds of exercise trackers count steps, so it's easier than ever to chart your walking progress. The average health-conscious American walks roughly 4,500 steps each day,[31] but there are many who do more; for example, Amish adults in the United States and the Toba hunters of Argentina walk more than 15,000 steps a day.[32, 33]

## ISABEL BEAT DIABETES IN HER BACKYARD

Isabel is a real-estate agent in her early 40s with a son in middle school and a daughter in high school. Her typical day is quite hectic, with a morning rush to get the kids ready for school before she gets out of the house around 9:00 a.m. to show clients different properties. Her day is spent driving around town, with no fixed time for lunch, so she had gotten into the habit of snacking every hour or two from morning to dinner. Between her husband's job, her work, and the kids' after-school activities, the family would typically get together after 9:00 p.m. to share ice cream or dessert.

For the last four or five years, at her annual physical checkup, Isabel's doctor had been telling her to eat healthy and be more active. But she did not understand that this advice was actually a warning until last year (2019), when her doctor told her that she has diabetes. He gave her a choice: start medication now or do an intensive lifestyle intervention. Isabel didn't want to take medication, so she thought she could eat less and move a little more. She joined a gym, spent some money on gym outfits and new shoes, bought a bunch of healthy snacks, and started to skip her breakfast two or three times a week. She spent the next year doing 45-minute workouts a day at the gym, including resistance training for two of the days and aerobics the rest of the time.

When she went for her annual checkup in January 2020, she thought her doctor would be happy. But his reaction was the opposite. Her doctor was very concerned. Her fasting blood glucose was above 160 mg/dL, her HbA1c was 8.1, her total cholesterol was at 290 (healthy is <200) and her blood pressure had reached 140/90. This time Isabel didn't get a choice: she was given the medication metformin and the doctor told her that she was a walking time bomb for heart disease.

Isabel heard about our study and signed up that same week. She chose to start on a 10-hour IF along with the metformin. Her doctor was a little concerned about her not eating for 14 hours but asked her to call the doctor's office if something went wrong.

It took a few weeks to adjust her routine completely, but Isabel was determined. She would send the kids to school and then have a big breakfast at 8:00 a.m. before heading out the door. She would pack a small salad with tofu for lunch and be back for dinner with the family at 6:00 p.m. By Week 4, she had figured out she needed more complex carbs, healthy fats, and protein to reduce her hunger pangs.

During Week 5, the COVID-19 pandemic hit. The gym was shut down. Isabel found herself stuck at home, completely sedentary and stressed out. She decided to walk in the backyard and around the block. She would walk at least 10,000 steps every day. Walking calmed her down amid the pandemic stress. It also improved her sleep quality. Since she was walking outdoors and getting enough daylight, it also uplifted her mood.

The 10-hour IF, a better diet, and 10,000 steps became her new normal, and by Week 6, her weight began to come down. By the end of three months, when she came back for her labs, her fasting blood glucose was 150, her HbA1c was down to 7.1, her blood pressure was down to 135/80. Even her cholesterol came down a bit to 265. We were thrilled to see her results.

Outside of the study, Isabel continued for another three months and her numbers got even better. She lost a total of 16 pounds, her morning fasting glucose was at 127, her HbA1c was at 6.5, her blood pressure was 130/80, and her cholesterol was 245. Best of all, her doctor cut her metformin prescription in half.

# WHEN TO EXERCISE

There are certain times of the day when exercise is more beneficial for boosting your circadian rhythm and reversing diabetes. However, any daily exercise is better than no exercise, even at a suboptimal window of opportunity. There are benefits to many choices, so choose the one that works best for you and your family.

## EXERCISE IN THE MORNING

The conventional wisdom is that you should eat before any physical activity. This is not always true. If you have fasted for 10 to 12 hours before your morning walk, run, or bike ride, you will likely tap into your stored body fat for energy during your exercise. Your muscles will spend more energy, using even more fat as the energy source, literally melting away even more body fat. And the more muscle you have, the more calories you'll burn throughout the day and the leaner and healthier you'll be.

Early morning is a great time to get outside and start moving with an aerobic activity. A brisk walk, or any outdoor activity in the presence of bright daylight, is an excellent way to synchronize the brain clock. It is also an important mechanism for maintaining and enhancing brain function. First, it will improve your mood for the rest of the day. Also, exercise stimulates new brain cell production,[34] and aids your ability to make new neuronal connections for deeper learning and more memory.

It doesn't matter whether you wait until sunrise to begin your morning activity. You can start anywhere from 30 minutes to 2 hours before or after sunrise. If you exercise in a gym or at home in the morning, find a spot that is next to a large glass window or under bright light.

As long as you are dressed properly for the weather, you can take a morning walk throughout most of the year, unless there is a weather advisory. In fact, exercising in cold air imparts some additional health benefits. Cold air activates the brown fat or converts the white fat to beige fat.[35] Brown fat is rich in mitochondria, the energy currency of any cell. More mitochondria mean that fat cells have more capacity to burn off. Additionally, body fat is burned to warm up the body during cold-air workouts. As a result, you can simply burn some fat by being exposed to cold temperatures.[36]

Some people with diabetes may be prone to increase their blood sugar level if they do strenuous aerobic exercise such as rowing, spinning, or jogging before breakfast. This phenomenon may be partly due to excess amounts of the stress hormone cortisol. Typically, cortisol levels peak an hour after we get out of bed. Exercise further boosts cortisol. High cortisol levels can trigger the body to release some sugar into the blood or prevent the muscles from absorbing glucose from the blood.[37] If you are exerting yourself to the point where your heart is beating faster, which is the goal during exercise, then you may be spiking your cortisol and inadvertently increasing your blood sugar levels.

You can test if morning exercise is right for you by taking a blood glucose reading in the morning before you start exercising and again right after you finish your exercise. If your blood glucose shoots up by 30 mg/dL (say from 120 to 150 mg/dL) or higher, then you need to take your intensity down a notch. You will get more benefit from a brisk walk: otherwise, your blood glucose will increase even further after eating breakfast. If this is the case for you, move your strenuous aerobic exercise to either after your breakfast or to the afternoon/evening.

## EXERCISE IN LATE AFTERNOON

Another great time for physical activity is at dusk or in the late afternoon,[38] starting from 3:00 p.m. to dinnertime. This is when muscle tone begins to rise, so it's the best time for strength training, including weight lifting, or vigorous aerobic exercise like spinning. It's also a great time to work on your yoga practice. Yoga requires flexibility, and your joints are looser and the body warmer in the afternoon/early evening.

Late-afternoon or early evening exercise has two practical benefits that directly influence diabetes risk. Exercise is known to reduce appetite,[39] so afternoon exercise not only helps burn some calories but can also help reduce hunger at dinnertime, so you may eat less. Exercise also helps the muscles take up more glucose in a mechanism that does not depend on insulin.[40] As insulin production and release gradually decline through the evening, insulin alone may not be sufficient to prevent your blood glucose levels from shooting up beyond the healthy range. As little as 15 minutes of evening exercise will boost your muscles' ability to absorb some blood glucose and keep it within a healthy range.

The lungs and heart are both muscles that have a circadian variation. That is, we have a relatively higher heart rate and heavier breathing during the day, and both slow down at night. The higher heart rate and breathing help distribute oxygen and nutrients throughout the body, including to the muscles during the day, priming us for physical activity. At night the muscles don't need the same levels of nutrients and oxygen as they do during the day. This may be one reason why heart rate and breathing slow down at night, which helps the body cool down so we can sleep better.

Some people worry that if they exercise in the early evening they will compress the amount of time they have between dinner and sleep. Let's say you're working a 9:00 a.m. to 5:00 p.m. job and you exercise after work and then you have dinner. Now you're pushing dinner to 7:30 or 8:00 p.m. That's okay, because exercise absolves some sins: the positive benefits of exercise outweigh a lost hour or two of IF (you'll learn more about this at the end of the chapter).

## EXERCISE AFTER DINNER

If you have been diagnosed with diabetes, evening exercise is your best option, because it has its own set of specific benefits that affect your circadian code for metabolism and maintaining blood sugar levels. Physical activity increases the demand for glucose, and muscles can soak up a good amount of blood glucose, thereby reducing the blood glucose spike after an evening meal so that you will be in a normal physiological range.

After dinner, mild physical activity, like an evening walk or doing chores in the house, helps digestion by moving the food along the digestive tract and by reducing the chance of acid reflux or heartburn. Since the insulin release and subsequent action on blood glucose regulation decline in the evening,[41,42] any physical activity in the evening is like taking a diabetes pill to reduce blood sugar. If you can create the ritual of taking a walk or doing some moderate exercise after dinner, it may also reduce your urge for a late-night snack because you will be busy and out of the kitchen.

Yet not all exercise at night is a good idea. It's best to do your extreme activity or high-intensity exercise before dinner. Late-night exercise in a gym or on a treadmill can increase cortisol to morning levels and delay the nightly rise of melatonin. Intense exercise also raises body temperature and heart rate. All these factors interfere with your ability to go to sleep. You may be resetting your clock by sending a signal that it's earlier in the day. This may be a reason why some (not all) people who exercise late at night also go to bed after midnight. If late night is the only time you can exercise, taking a shower before bedtime can help your body cool down, which will help you get to sleep.

## COMBINE INTERMITTENT FASTING WITH EXERCISE

Our research found three substantial benefits related to combining diet and exercise. The first improvement was in muscle mass. We assumed that fasting for 14 to 16 hours would break down mice muscles and we would see a reduction in muscle mass. Actually, we found the exact opposite. When mice ate for only 12 hours, we never saw a reduction in muscle mass. In fact, only fat mass was reduced. If the mice ate a healthy diet within an 8- to 10-hour window, they gradually increased their muscle mass, and after 36 weeks they had 10 to 15 percent more muscle mass than mice that ate whenever they wanted.[43]

We also know that many genes that are involved in repairing muscle and growing muscle are circadian, with a peak production during the day. These genes are directly under the instruction of both a circadian clock and the feeding–fasting cycle. In our lab, we found that muscle repair and rejuvenation genes in mice got a double boost from having a healthy circadian clock and also in having a clear feeding–fasting cycle. This might explain why they gained more muscle mass.

One improvement we saw in the IF mice was an increase in the capacity for endurance exercise. That is, when we start such long physical activity, the body initially taps into the readily available sugar as an energy source, and when the glucose or glycogen is depleted, we "hit the wall." The brain and body get exhausted of energy and we cannot run any longer. But endurance training helps the muscles with two hugely beneficial metabolic adaptations. First, muscle learns to absorb more glucose from the blood when food is available so that there is a larger store of glucose and glycogen to use during endurance training. Second, it learns to adapt to an alternate energy source when all the stored glycogen is used up. When this happens, the muscle switches to using stored fat as its energy source. The fat is converted to ketone bodies, and this simple carbon source is used as fuel for the extra miles. Combining time-restricted eating with exercising for more than an hour gives the body double benefits. IF boosts the signals for muscle repair and regeneration to help sustain or build muscle mass, and increased physical activity helps soak up more glucose from the bloodstream into muscle, so the extra glucose is diverted from the liver, where it was going to be stored as fat.

We have also seen improvement when we link motor coordination and IF. We found that mice following a restricted eating pattern had increased motor coordination. In my lab, we put mice in a rotating drum, where they had to balance themselves. We found that if they ate for 8 to 10 hours, they could stay on the drum 20 percent longer.

Intermittent fasting can be further boosted when combined with timed exercise. For instance, people who exercise on a regular basis report they feel less hungry the rest of the day,[44] making a 10-hour IF more manageable. The reason is that exercise reduces the hunger hormone ghrelin and increases the satiety hormones, which are also under circadian control. Intense exercise has a stronger effect on hunger compared to moderate exercise.

## THE EXERCISE-FOR-IF SWAP

If you can't follow your daily eating routine, crank up your exercise to keep you on track for reversing diabetes. As discussed in the previous chapter, during the overnight fast, the body slowly burns stored carbs (glycogen) before tapping into the carbs already stored as body fat. One of the benefits of IF comes from this slow fat-burning. When you eat over a longer window, the body does not get enough fasting time to burn the stored carbs. This is where exercise comes in handy. When you exercise, the body burns off a goodly amount of readily available sugar and stored carbohydrates. Something as simple as brisk walking for an hour can burn off the equivalent of 50 to 75 grams of carbs. Running for the same time can double the burn.

Another reason to make this swap is that on non-IF days, your body is digesting food and absorbing sugar over many extra hours. Since exercise can help your muscles better absorb glucose after a meal, you can add a layer of control over your blood glucose by exercising more on the non-IF days. Taking a brisk walk or doing some chores at home after a later night meal can help your digestion and reduce the risk of heartburn. The later exercise and a shower will also help you sleep better, because otherwise the undigested food would keep you awake.

## WHAT'S NEXT

Speaking of sleep, in the next chapter I explain the circadian reasons why both getting good sleep every night and limiting exposure to bright light in the evening can positively affect your blood sugar.

## CHAPTER 8

# Optimize Sleep and Light Exposure

There is an emerging consensus that sleeping less or having disrupted sleep affects brain function, imbalances the hormones, and increases inflammation. All these factors can negatively affect your blood glucose. First, fewer than 6 hours of nightly sleep is correlated with an increased risk for developing prediabetes, diabetes, and the sinister friends of diabetes (including hypertension, obesity, and heart diseases).[1] In a landmark study by Professor Eve van Cauter, 11 healthy men who typically slept for 8 hours each night were limited to only 4 hours every night for six days, followed by 12 hours of sleep for the next six days. After five days of each type of sleep, the men were tested to see how their bodies responded to glucose. The results showed rather strikingly that sleeping less reduces the body's ability to bring down blood glucose levels after drinking a glass of glucose water—as if the person is almost diabetic. When the same men in the study had slept well, their blood glucose control returned to normal. It was also learned that when the men had slept longer, they achieved recovery sleep that reversed the damage done during the first half of the experiment.[2] This result has been repeated several times in other studies, all of which led to the same conclusion: sleeping fewer than 6 hours can predispose someone to prediabetes.

We also know that a sleep-deprived brain is a diabetic brain. Almost 30 years ago, scientists put sleep-deprived people under brain-imaging tests to assess how the brain uses glucose. The researchers were hoping to find that the brain would go into overdrive to stay awake and thereby would use more glucose. But surprisingly, the scientists found that many brain regions did not increase their glucose consumption when there were more waking hours. Instead, a few brain regions reduced their glucose usage,[3] because the glucose could not get inside the brain cells. Just like in diabetes, the blood glucose cannot enter the brain cells and instead remains in the blood, raising the blood glucose level. This means that certain parts of the brain don't get their daily dose of energy when we stay awake for too many hours each day.

This study triggered a series of other studies on the effect of sleep deprivation on brain function. Now we know that sleep deprivation literally rewires the brain,[4,5] and it thwarts the detoxification that is supposed to happen during a good night's sleep.[6,7] These changes may start a cascade of events leading to increased risk for diabetes. For example, sleep deprivation hyperactivates a certain brain region involved in food cravings,[8] triggering the person to eat foods that can affect blood glucose, like ultra-processed foods that are high in simple sugars.

As the brain is the master regulator of almost all hormones in the body, sleep loss changes the level or the timing of every major hormone.[9] For example, it affects the presence of melatonin, the sleep hormone. Just like melatonin puts the brain to sleep, it also makes your pancreas sleep. When you have a good night of restful sleep and wake up without an alarm clock, you arise with lower levels of melatonin in the morning. However, if you have a poor night's sleep, or you need to wake up in the morning to an alarm clock, your brain will still be cranking out melatonin, and it may take a few more hours before it starts to come down. After a night of insufficient sleep, your higher morning melatonin level can prevent your pancreas from releasing enough insulin to deal with breakfast, leading to a start of the day with increased blood sugar.

A sleep-deprived brain also craves excessive calories that it does not need, resulting in weight gain.[10] Sleep deprivation directly affects the hunger and satiety hormones ghrelin and leptin, both of which have a circadian nature. Ghrelin is produced in the stomach whenever the stomach is empty, and it is the signal to the brain to feel hunger. Leptin is produced in the fat cells and signals the brain that you are full. However, poor sleep patterns disrupt these signals and make a person more prone to overeating because the brain isn't getting either of these two messages. Sleep loss also reduces leptin production, and the imbalance created between leptin and ghrelin may explain why after a sleepless night, the gut craves a bigger carbohydrate-heavy breakfast in the morning,[11] which affects the blood sugar.

There are other mechanisms that cause the body to overeat when we don't have enough sleep. We think the reason is that the brain wants to ensure we have enough calories to cover activity during those hours. But in controlled studies, participants who reduced their sleep from 8 hours to 5 hours consistently overate more calories than what would be required to fuel a few extra hours of wakefulness. At the same time, the stress hormone cortisol stays high in the evening after just one night of less sleep.[12] Excess cortisol is known to reduce the effect of insulin, so your blood glucose level may rise the following day, reaching a peak the next evening, when it really should be at its lowest point of the day.

Poor sleep can also cause changes in the immune system. Inflammation in the body is supposed to reduce during sleep. If you don't sleep long enough, the inflammation doesn't have time to subside. Inflammation or unnecessary activation of the immune system contributes to diabetes and its complications, including heart diseases. While this connection has been known for many years, the mechanism is only beginning to be clear. It seems that when we have a good night's sleep and wake up normally, the brain produces the hormone hypocretin, which acts as a quality control for the bone marrow. With the correct amount of hypocretin, only the right type of immune cells from the bone marrow are produced.[13] But with poor sleep, these immune cells do not fully mature and may overreact in response to the usual housekeeping functions of defending the body against pathological agents and thereby increase inflammation. This inflammation can exacerbate the effects of diabetes by increasing the risk for heart diseases. Other studies have shown that too much or too little sleep is related to higher levels of inflammation, which in turn may contribute to elevated blood glucose.[14]

Many people who are overweight and/or diabetic also have sleep apnea, which is one of the major causes of sleep deprivation. It occurs when you have a blockage or obstruction in the nasal cavity or throat or have a floppy tongue that obstructs your airways either partially or completely during the night. The obstructions deprive the brain and the body of oxygen and cause an automatic response that wakes up a person just enough to breathe again, although maybe not to wake to the point of consciousness. These upsets can occur all night long, yet people with sleep apnea very often have no clue. Instead, they'll wake up in the morning without feeling refreshed. Other subtle clues include waking up with a dry mouth or having to repeatedly use the bathroom in the middle of the night.

Some people with sleep apnea snore—but not all of them. And not all snoring is considered to be sleep apnea. Your partner might be a better detective than you in determining if you are suffering from sleep apnea. For example, if you have been told that you hold your breath during the night, you may have sleep apnea.

Sleep apnea affects not only the quality and quantity of a person's sleep but also one's brain health. Cognitive problems, such as deficits in memory, attention, and visual abilities, frequently accompany obstructive sleep apnea. It is also a major risk factor for diabetes, heart disease, and stroke, since as many as two-thirds of people with underlying sleep apnea have one of these conditions.[15,16]

A sleep study can help you determine if you are suffering from sleep apnea. The standard treatment for sleep apnea is a device referred to as a CPAP (continuous positive airway pressure), which is prescribed by a doctor; trained medical staff guide you on how to use the machine. It is a mask that you wear over your nose and mouth that is hooked up to a machine to make sure you have a constant supply of air. There are other devices and apps that can monitor oxygen intake as well. The good news is that those who are compliant with the use of CPAP are more likely to improve their blood glucose regulation during their sleep,[17] setting themselves up for better glucose regulation the following day.

## SLEEP LETS THE WHOLE BODY RESET

Sleep is not a shutting down of bodily functions; instead, a whole different assortment of essential bodily functions takes place that cannot happen when we are awake. Many of these functions are meant to repair and restore the cells, because every day, the body battles with stressors that create cellular damage. Sleeping less or having frequently disrupted sleep does a lot of harm to the body by not letting it repair itself well.

At night, we aren't just making necessary repairs to the body; the brain is also busy consolidating memories and sending out instructions to prepare us for the next round of activity. The changes that happen at night are absolutely critical to how we feel the next day. That's why when we are in good health and have the right amount of sleep, we wake up feeling refreshed. Adults with poor sleep habits are more likely to develop anxiety and depression, and seniors may experience memory impairment.[18,19]

Waking up with joint pain may be a sign that you did not get a good night's sleep for several days in a row. You might find that if you sleep fewer than 6 hours a night for three or four nights, when you wake up your joints are stiff or you might have a pain in your knee. However, if you can get onto a better sleep schedule, you may find that after a week or two of restful sleep, those pains go away without any medication, without any exercise, and without changing your diet.

To access the benefits of good sleep, you have to achieve a prescribed number of hours of sleep. From tracking a million individuals, researchers have identified a pattern, known as the U curve of sleep and longevity.[20] That is, people who consistently sleep too little are more likely to die earlier than those who get the full 7 hours of sleep each night.

Similarly, people who sleep as much as 10 or 11 hours are likely to live shorter lives. The majority of people who had an ideal body mass index (BMI)—a standard health measurement that tracks a healthy weight-to-height ratio—were also shown to sleep 7 hours a night. The bottom line is that too much or too little sleep can be detrimental.

---

**LOOK CLOSELY AT YOUR SLEEP ROUTINE**

One way to see if you are in this sweet spot of the U curve is to track your sleep habits. You can use the chart on page 85 to fill in when you go to sleep and wake up, or you can use the myCircadianClock app (available at myCircadianClock.org), or any wearable sleep tracker, smartwatch, or even your mobile phone. The more you know about your sleep patterns, the easier they are to correct.

---

## THE PERFECT AMOUNT OF SLEEP

As soon as we wake up, the SCN begins keeping track of our wakeful time. For every hour we stay awake, we later have to sleep 20 to 30 minutes. In the evening, the organs' unique clocks synchronize with one another to create the perfect condition for sleep. The pineal gland inside the brain begins to produce the sleep hormone melatonin. At the same time, the heart clock instructs the heart rate to slow down, and the SCN instructs the body to cool down. Then, when the timing is right and the lights are low, you go to sleep.

Every night, adults should give themselves 8 consecutive hours of "sleep opportunity," and children should have 10 hours of the same. That opportunity includes getting into bed, settling down, then falling asleep. Children should be sleeping for at least 9 hours a night; adults should sleep for no fewer than 7 hours.[21,22]

A sleep debt is the difference between the amount of sleep you should be getting and the amount you actually get. So, if you slept for 6½ hours last night, you're beginning your day with 30 minutes of sleep debt. When you go to sleep the following night, you first repay this debt from the previous night. That means that even if you sleep 7 hours on the second night, it counts only as sleeping for 6½—again. That's one of the reasons why we often sleep late on weekends: it's the body's way of repaying our entire sleep debt.

Having sleep debt increases the propensity to sleep, while circadian rhythm instructs when to sleep. For instance, if you are awake for two days, you have too much sleep debt to unload in a single night. You'll go to sleep, but your circadian clock won't allow you to sleep continuously for 16 hours. The first night you might sleep for 8, 9, or maybe 10 hours, then the circadian drive kicks in to wake you up. The next day you're still sleepy because the clock is telling the brain it's time to stay awake, but the sleep debt is telling the brain that you ought to go back to sleep. That conflict goes on into the following night, again, when you'll sleep a little longer until you catch up.

### NAPPING HELPS REPAY A SLEEP DEBT

A short nap during the day is one way to repay your sleep debt. If you had a sleep debt of 2 hours during the workweek, and you took a long Saturday afternoon nap, it's possible to repay that debt in one nap. But be careful not to sleep too long: a long afternoon nap will dissipate some of the sleep pressure that was building up, but the longer you sleep in the afternoon, the more difficult you may find it is to fall asleep when you want to later that night.

## HOW LONG SHOULD YOU SLEEP?

Recommended Hours of Sleep Across the Lifespan: Chronic Insufficient Sleep in Childhood Can Increase the Risk for Diabetes in Adulthood.*

| | | HOURS OF SLEEP | | MINUTES IT TAKES TO FALL ASLEEP | | NO. OF TIMES WAKING UP FOR LIFE | |
| --- | --- | --- | --- | --- | --- | --- | --- |
| | Age | Ideal | Not recommended | Normal | Talk to your doctor | Normal | Talk to your doctor |
| NEWBORNS | 0-3 mths. | 14-17 hrs. | <11 or >19 hrs. | 0-30 mins. | >45 mins. | 3+ times | |
| INFANTS | 4-11 mths. | 12-15 hrs. | <10 or >18 hrs. | 0-30 mins. | >45 mins. | 3+ times | |
| TODDLERS | 1-2 yrs. | 11-14 hrs. | <9 or >17 hrs. | 0-30 mins. | >45 mins. | 1 | >4 |
| PRE-SCHOOLERS | 3-5 yrs. | 10-13 hrs. | <8 or >16 hrs. | 0-30 mins. | >45 mins. | 1 | >4 |
| SCHOOL-AGED CHILDREN | 6-13 yrs. | 9-11 hrs. | <7 or >15 hrs. | 0-30 mins. | >45 mins. | 1 | >4 |
| TEENAGERS | 14-17 yrs. | 8-10 hrs. | <7 or >13 hrs. | 0-30 mins. | >45 mins. | 1 | >4 |
| ADULTS | 18-64 yrs. | 7-9 hrs. | <6 or >10 hrs. | 0-30 mins. | >45 mins. | 1 | >4 |
| OLDER ADULTS | >65 yrs. | 7-8 hrs. | <6 or >10 hrs. | 0-30 mins. | >60 mins. | 2 | >4 |

(*M. Ohayon et al., "National Sleep Foundation's Sleep Quality Recommendations: First Report," Sleep Health 3, no. 1 (2017):, 6–19)

## ARE YOU SLEEPING WELL?

Ask yourself the following three questions to get a clear picture of your sleep quality.

### QUESTION 1: WHEN DO YOU GO TO BED, AND HOW LONG DOES IT TAKE FOR YOU TO FALL ASLEEP?

First, let's lower the bar a bit. Most people do not shut off the lights and fall asleep immediately. An average person who has good sleep habits should be able to fall asleep within 20 minutes of getting into bed and shutting off the lights. During this 20-minute period there should be nothing else between you and sleep. No book. No phone. No light.

If you struggle to fall asleep and you're in bed for more than 30 minutes, turning and tossing, that's a sign you have difficulty getting to sleep. This is the definition of insomnia: difficulty falling asleep.

The main culprits for insomnia are:

- Worry: This increases production of the stress hormone cortisol, which is meant to keep us awake.

- Too much food: This keeps the core body temperature too high for sleep.

- Too little physical activity: This reduces the production of the muscle hormone that promotes sleep.

- Too much time spent in bright light in the evening: this reduces melatonin production.

### QUESTION 2: HOW MANY TIMES DO YOU WAKE UP DURING THE NIGHT?

Fragmented sleep is defined as waking up more than once during the night for at least a few minutes, to the point where it's difficult to go back to sleep. This type of sleep is not optimal because the brain registers only the time you sleep, and it responds as if it isn't getting any sleep at all during these periods of fragmented sleep. For instance, if you were in bed for 8 hours but woke up three or four times, then your brain might register only 4 or 5 hours of actual sleep. Even if you woke up for only 10 or 15 minutes each time, it takes additional time to get back to that deep sleep phase, and you miss out on this continuous, uninterrupted sleep.

As we age, sleep becomes more fragile, and it is common to experience fragmented sleep. The arousal threshold decreases with age, so we wake up to simple noises or disturbances. However, it is possible to sleep through the night without fragmented sleep, especially if you align your sleep time with your circadian code.

The main causes of fragmented sleep are:

- Dehydration
- Ambient temperature being too hot or cold
- Acid reflux caused by eating too late in the evening
- Sleeping with a person/pet who wakes up at night
- Snoring/sleep apnea
- Other noises

## QUESTION 3: DO YOU FEEL RESTED WHEN YOU WAKE UP IN THE MORNING?

If you need to wake up to an alarm clock, or if you wake up feeling sleepy or foggy, then you aren't waking up feeling rested, and it's likely you did not get enough sleep. The main causes of insufficient sleep relate to the difficulty of falling asleep or fragmented sleep. Other causes include:

- Sleep debt from previous days. If you habitually sleep for 7 hours and slept only 6 hours each night for the previous three nights, then sleeping 7 or 8 hours won't be enough and you may not feel fully rested in the morning.

- Sleep apnea (see page 168).

- Lights or sounds during sleep. Although you may not wake up, light in the room or ambient noise may be disturbing your sleep. You may not wake up, but you won't feel rested in the morning.

## FIX YOUR SLEEP WITH INTERMITTENT FASTING

The types of foods you eat and when you eat them can positively affect your sleep. According to the Sleep Foundation, eating certain foods a few times each week has shown promising benefits. For example, a fatty fish like salmon[23] or nuts like walnuts[24] contain important vitamins, including vitamin D and zinc, which are linked with better sleep. And the typical foods associated with a Mediterranean diet (see page 217), have been associated with promoting better sleep.[25]

Drinking alcohol before bed has a different effect on sleep when compared to eating sweets, yet it is just as disruptive. In an oxymoronic way, alcoholic beverages dehydrate you, and the more you drink before bedtime, the thirstier you will be in the middle of the night. So, while some people may use a late-night drink to fall asleep, they generally have difficulty staying asleep. Once you are used to having a good night's sleep, having that glass of wine at night will seem less appealing, which is good, because alcohol is not recommended for those with a risk for diabetes. One man in our study group used to have three or four cocktails after dinner. When he started cutting down on his alcohol, he found that he was sleeping better. After a while, he gave up his cocktails entirely. He told me, "It's not that I don't enjoy a cocktail anymore, I just really like my good night's sleep better."

Once you adopt IF, your sleep is likely to improve, and once your sleep improves, it will also help you have better control over what and when you eat. By adopting IF you can turn the vicious cycle of bad sleep and bad food choices into one of good sleep and good food choices. In my lab, we have found that a 10-hour eating window offers the most benefits. Following this regimen, our mice achieved a cooler body temperature during sleep and slept more soundly. While they didn't sleep longer than mice that eat randomly, the electrical recordings of their brain activity showed that their sleep was deeper and perhaps more restful (we cannot ask a mouse if it slept well). We don't know the reasons for this; we believe that the basic sleep drive does not change under IF, but that IF puts the mice into deeper sleep.

Through our app, myCircadianClock, we have observed that many people doing a 10-hour IF have reported substantial improvement in their sleep. In fact, some of them continue to do IF, not for weight loss or diabetes control but to sleep better at night.[26] In a 2020 study of people with metabolic syndrome, we found that almost everyone in the study also reported at least one improvement in sleep: they slept longer, slept deeper, or felt they had a more restful sleep at night.[27]

We also know that eating late at night affects one's sleep. This late-night habit interferes with both falling asleep and maintaining deep sleep. In order to fall asleep, the core body temperature must cool down by almost 1°F. But when we eat, the core body temperature actually goes up as blood rushes to the gut to help digest and absorb nutrients. Therefore, eating late at night prevents people from getting into a deep sleep. To have a good night's sleep, you should have your last meal 2 to 4 hours before going to bed, so as to ensure that the body is able to cool down.

Even a sleepy brain may work better without adding food to the mix for hours at a time. Research in Mark Mattson's lab at the National Institutes of Health has shown that mice that undergo a longer fasting period have better brain function, as keeping to a restricted eating time strengthens the connections or synapses between the brain cells.[28] We believe that a stronger connection between those neurons means the human brain can think better and remember better, regardless of how rested we are.

> **DRINKING WATER AT NIGHT ISN'T A PROBLEM**
>
> I always have a glass of water next to my bed. Some people think that if they drink water in the middle of the night, then they're going to wake up again. In reality, you're not drinking more than a few ounces. In fact, ignoring your thirst is far worse: a dry throat is the reason you probably woke up in the first place.

## BRIGHT LIGHT AT NIGHT ENABLES BAD HABITS

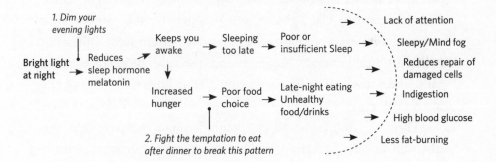

Bright light at night reduces your ability to make melatonin, which ultimately can limit your sleep. Sleeping less can increase hunger, and a sleepy brain makes it difficult to make the right food choices. Both bad sleep and late-night eating increase your risk for indigestion, allow damaged cells to accumulate in your organs, reduce the fat-burning process, and can increase blood glucose. You can break this cycle by (1) dimming your lights for 2 to 3 hours before bedtime, and (2) adopting an IF whereby you stop eating 2 to 3 hours before bedtime.

## MANAGING LIGHT EXPOSURE CAN FIX WHEN AND HOW WE SLEEP

Everyone knows it is hard to fall asleep in a brightly lit room, and it is easy to doze off in a dimly lit room (such as a classroom or your TV room). The reason is not simply the brightness of the light. My research has revealed how different colors of light, particularly blue light, affect the circadian clock, which then affects a person's mood and sleep. These disruptions can increase your risk for developing diabetes.[29]

Scientists have known for a long time that many blind people and blind animals cannot see the world around them, yet they can sense when they are in bright light. In fact, they can even reset their circadian clock and sleep–wake cycle with the change of seasons, when the sun is at a different angle in the sky, or if they travel from one time zone to another. In 2001, I was on a research team that discovered that a special blue light sensor in our eyes (and in the eyes of many animals), called melanopsin, is responsible for the nonvisual function of interpreting light. Ever since then, researchers like me have been working to determine how melanopsin operates. We have found that this light sensor is most sensitive to blue light and less sensitive to red or orange light. It also requires exposure to several minutes of bright light to be fully activated. Once activated, though, it sends the light information to the brain, where it is used for many functions, including synchronizing our circadian clocks.

When our ancestors lived in a world without electrical light, the light from flickering candles or firelight was enough to see what's around at night, but not enough to activate the melanopsin. The relative darkness sent their brain's clock a signal that it was nighttime, and their melatonin levels would rise to make them fall asleep around 9:00 or 10:00 p.m. In the morning, when those ancestors woke up with the sunrise and walked into the bright daylight (which is a rich source of blue light), they would fully activate their melanopsin, and the brain clock would receive the signal to suppress melatonin and lift their mood.

One downside of our modern lifestyle is that the extra light we are exposed to at night is not good for maintaining a strong circadian rhythm. Bright lights and bright screens at night continue to activate the melanopsin sensor, which in turn reduces melatonin production. This is one reason why we cannot fall asleep easily after watching television or working at a computer screen at night. And during the day, we spend most of our time indoors now. Dim indoor lighting in the morning does not fully suppress the melatonin, nor does it naturally lift our mood; it confuses the brain's circadian clock.

In order to resync the brain's clock to achieve better sleep and control blood glucose, we have to make conscious changes to how we manage our light sources. These changes aren't drastic; all you need to do is step outside every day to get at least 30 minutes of bright daylight exposure, preferably in the morning before breakfast. Although we don't know exactly how the mechanism works, studies have shown that exposure to bright daylight, or even to blue-enriched white light (the light you may get from "cool white" LED lights), can increase your nightly melatonin level, which helps with falling asleep and staying asleep.[30,31] Spending the day in sun-drenched rooms can help, but getting outside is still better.

In addition to increasing your exposure to bright daylight, you need to reduce the amount of blue-light exposure during the evening. Clinical studies have shown that reducing blue-light exposure improves sleep.[32] Digital screens are a significant source of such blue light, and we typically spend more than 8 hours a day looking at them. Luckily, there are now apps for our smartphones and computer screens that can change the brightness and color of a traditional blue-light screen to a slightly orange-looking screen that is lower in blue light. This change in color can be programmed to occur automatically each day, synced with the time you want to go to sleep. Additionally, almost every new smartphone, laptop, and tablet has a built-in function to set the time at which the screen brightness or color will change, automatically going into sleep mode. For smartphones, Apple calls this their Night Shift feature and Samsung's is called Dark mode (or Night mode on older phones). To set it, all you need to do is enter the start time for 2 hours before your preferred sleep and wake times, and the app takes care of the rest, reducing the blue light of the screen to transform it from a bright white to an orange glow.

Many new televisions also include this technology. Features such as Samsung's Eye Saver Mode gradually changes the color and reduces the blue light on its TV screens. Your eyes adapt slowly, so that you won't even notice the change in color as it's happening. If you don't want to run out and buy a new television, though, there are add-on products that can transform your current one. For example, DriftTV is a small device that connects to your television through an HDMI input: use it to adjust the percentage of blue light from the screen. For example, you can set a DriftTV to remove 50 percent (or any percentage in increments of 10) of all blue light over a period of 1 hour. That way, the transition is seamless and virtually unnoticeable.

These changes are small but significant. What is so sneaky about melanopsin is that we don't feel any change occurring, but the circadian clock, sleep, and mood respond to these changes in a profound way. It's easy enough to give it a try.

We can also pay attention to the type of light that we are exposed to in the evening. I'm not suggesting you spend the evenings in a dark room until you go to bed. There are many techniques and products, though, that can help reduce your exposure to other types of blue light. For instance, in the evenings, you can shut off overhead lights and use table lamps instead. For rooms like the kitchen or bathroom, dimmer switches will help you easily reduce ambient overhead light. Timers can be programmed to turn off or on lights at different times of the day. These strategies are easy fixes to reduce your light exposure at night.

Even dim light from innocuous sources like the lights on small home electronics (like bedside alarm clocks) can compromise your sleep and circadian rhythm. Many people are sensitive to dim light, and they sleep better with an eye mask or in a completely dark room in which every possible light source is covered. And if you wake up in the middle of the night to get a drink of water or go to the bathroom, turning on a light makes it infinitely harder to fall back asleep, so try to keep any nightlights to a minimum. Place a glass of water next to your bed, which will save you the trip to the kitchen. Or, if you need to use the bathroom, here's where having your cell phone nearby comes in handy: use the flashlight feature to illuminate the floor to help you find your way.

If you have difficulty falling asleep, try wearing glasses that filter blue light for an hour or two before bedtime. Blocking that blue light can trigger earlier release of the sleep hormone melatonin. And as you've learned, with better sleep, you can better control your blood glucose. If you need to wear prescription glasses, look for blue light glasses that are oversize so that they can go over your prescription glasses.

## SUSAN MANAGES HER BLOOD SUGAR WITH A BLUE LIGHT HACK

My friend Susan has diabetes, and her morning readings for her fasting blood glucose are typically around 150 mg/dL, even with taking medications, doing IF, and following a healthy Mediterranean diet. She really wanted to lower the amount of medication she was taking, so we looked at other aspects of her lifestyle. When we were talking, we realized that she travels frequently for work, and on those nights away from home she has an especially hard time falling asleep. On the nights she is home, her typical bedtime was after midnight, yet she has to wake up around 6:00 a.m.

I suggested she try using blue-light-filtering glasses in the evening for a few hours after dinner, while she watched TV or was using her phone. She agreed, and we talked again the following week. Susan told me that adjustment was hard the first couple of days and it felt a little quirky to watch TV with them. But after the third day she hardly noticed the filter. And she realized that she was getting tired earlier in the evening and started going to bed around 10:30 p.m. That was great news, because she was getting at least $1^{1}/_{2}$ hours more sleep each night. The blue-light-filtering glasses made her sleepy earlier and made it easier for her to fall asleep.

We were so pleased with her progress that we agreed to check in two weeks later and have her take a fasting blood glucose reading. When we got together next, her three weeks straight of great sleep were paying off. Susan's IF program, combined with better sleep, helped her consistently reduce her fasting blood glucose below 130 mg/dL. This lower number is critical because it moved her out of the diabetes range and back to the prediabetes range. I suggested that she could take this information to her doctor so they could revisit her medication needs.

We realized that the blue-light-filtering glasses were integral to her success after she took her first trip and forgot to bring them with her. In her hotel, she went back to her old habit of falling asleep past midnight, and after a few nights her blood glucose level went right back up to 140 or 150. When she returned home, she started using the glasses again, and within a few days she reduced her fasting blood glucose by 10 to 20 points.

## STILL NOT SLEEPING?

If you've adjusted your nighttime light exposure and still are consistently not getting a good night's sleep, or if you are waking up at night, try the following techniques:

### TURN DOWN THE TEMPERATURE

The body has to cool down during nighttime to sleep. It's a good idea to reduce the temperature in your bedroom to 70°F or lower so that your skin feels cooler. When this happens, blood flows toward your skin to keep your skin warm. Since the blood is flowing away from the core of the body, the core body temperature can lower and you will fall asleep much easier.

If you cannot control the thermostat in your home, take a shower or a warm bath just before going to bed. Warm water also forces the blood flow toward your skin and away from the core.

Some people fall asleep, but after a few hours they wake up feeling hot. Experiment with your blankets to find what works best for you. If the blanket is not the culprit, think about your mattress. Foam mattresses are known to capture and retain heat. In the first few hours, the mattress helps you cool down, but after a few hours the foam can reflect the heat back to your body and warm you up.

## TURN THE SOUND UP, OR DOWN

In many cities, street sounds and emergency sirens make it difficult to fall asleep. Double- or triple-pane windows will cut out sounds to a great extent. For years, shift workers have used the hum of a fan blowing in their bedroom to suppress or block out disturbing noises. A more modern approach is a white-noise machine or app. These devices can make it easier to fall asleep and stay asleep by fighting noise with noise: the machine creates a wall of consistent sound that muffles any intruding noises that might engage your brain during sleep. Indeed, some people actually find white sound soothing, helping them to fall asleep. They put a radio or smartphone on a timer and play relaxing music at a low volume for a few minutes until they fall asleep.

For other people, like me, even small noises (like a noisy air conditioner or a partner who snores) can wake them up. This is where earplugs come in. When I travel, I always bring earplugs. Yet not all earplugs are created equal. Some are soft, some are hard, some are silicone, and some are like a sponge. You may have to try a few to find the type that's most comfortable for you. They have to fit your ear well, so that you don't have a sore ear canal in the morning. But once you find the right earplugs, you will experience a better night's sleep immediately: they make a huge difference.

## SNORING?

If you have been told that you snore, the easiest, least invasive fix is using a gentle saline spray or neti pot before bed. These are meant to cleanse and open up stuffy noses. The saline spray is safe for both adults and children to use every day.

Or, try a physical tool that keeps your nose open. There are two main types: ones that open your nostrils slightly wider, like a Breathe Right nasal strip; and ones that are inserted inside the nose to open the airway. By making breathing easier throughout the night they also allow you to take in more oxygen, which improves the quality of your sleep quite a lot. Sometimes, if I'm tired at the end of a long day of work, I will wear a Breathe Right strip on my nose as I'm driving home. My nose is chronically stuffy, and because I take in less oxygen during the day compared to other people, I get tired earlier. So I use my 30-minute commute to increase my oxygen intake and by the time I reach home, I'm really full of energy again.

If snoring continues even after these over-the-counter fixes, see an ear, nose, and throat specialist (ENT) or a pulmonary medicine sleep specialist.

## SLEEP MEDICATIONS

Sleep medications fall into two different categories. The first group is those that improve your ability to fall asleep, like Ambien (zolpidem), Lunesta (eszopiclone), and Restoril (temazepam). If you fall into the camp who need this type of drug, consider trying melatonin supplements first, as they can naturally reduce the time between going to bed and falling asleep.[33]

The second group of medications is for people who cannot stay asleep, or who wake up too many times throughout the night. These sleep medications, like Silenor (doxepin), help people with fragmented sleep get uninterrupted sleep, but some are so strong that in the morning people still experience sleepiness and brain fog. These medications help you fall asleep, but they don't help you wake up.

Sleep medications are not a permanent cure for sleep problems; when you get used to them, your brain relies on the medication to help you fall asleep. While effective, they also have significant drawbacks. Many studies have shown that the long-term use of sleep medications is associated with increased risk of Type 2 diabetes, heart disease, dementia, and cancer.[34] And if you are a frequent user of these medications, or have been taking sleep medication for a long time, it can take up to two weeks to try to fall asleep without them. Lastly, certain sleep medications have adverse side effects that mirror many of the complications of diabetes, including dizziness, light-headedness, headache, gastrointestinal problems, prolonged daytime drowsiness, severe allergic reactions, and daytime memory and performance problems.

## MELATONIN SUPPLEMENTATION

The sleep-promoting effect of melatonin supplementation has been known for almost five decades. We need melatonin to sleep. The body produces its own supply, but as we age, the pineal gland produces less melatonin at night. A 60-year-old produces one-half to one-third of the melatonin of a 10-year-old. Therefore, boosting nightly melatonin with a pill may be reasonable if you are having problems getting to sleep.

Try taking the melatonin supplement 2 to 3 hours before going to bed. However, be aware that melatonin can interfere with blood glucose regulation. The blood glucose naturally goes up after a meal and takes an hour or longer to come back to its normal level. Taking melatonin after a meal slows down that decline in blood glucose to the normal level. Therefore, it is a bad idea to take melatonin right after eating; instead, wait for at least an hour or two after a meal so that the melatonin doesn't interfere with your blood glucose level.

In many individuals, natural melatonin levels begin to rise 2 to 4 hours before their most frequent bedtime. If this is true for you, the best time to take melatonin is 2 hours before bedtime. This means that if you are planning on going to bed around 10:00 p.m., eat your dinner at 6:00 p.m. and take your melatonin at 8:00 p.m.

The effective dosing of melatonin seems to vary from person to person. Some people are very sensitive and a small, 1 mg dose may be more than enough, while other people take 5 mg to get better sleep.

## BEHAVIORAL TECHNIQUES FOR BETTER SLEEP

Here are some suggestions for lowering your stress about sleep, so that you can actually do it:

1. Don't stress about the time if you wake up in the middle of the night, so you don't have to look at your brightly lit watch, clock, or phone. The light from these devices will trigger your melanopsin. It really doesn't matter what time it is when you wake up in the middle of the night, and there's no benefit to starting to worry about not getting enough sleep. If you need an alarm clock to wake up at a certain time, that's fine: set it and cover it so that even those lights don't disturb your sleep.

2. Don't create stress near bedtime or worry that you will wake up late the next day—that's what alarm clocks are for. Relying on alarm clocks is not ideal, but as you are working on improving your circadian sleep rhythm, there is a place for them in your life. Instead of worrying that you won't wake up on time, try deep belly breathing to relax your body and mind.

3. Don't create stress about your last night's sleep and worry that you'll have the same bad experience again. You are in control of your sleep. By following the recommendations we've laid out in this chapter, you'll quite likely see your sleep improve, bit by bit, every night.

4. Don't stress about the number of hours you're currently sleeping. If you are feeling fine and restored the next day, you may not need as much sleep as others. But if you don't feel rested and refreshed in the morning, or if you feel sleepy during the late afternoon, try some of the tips in this chapter.

## THE BEST WAYS TO WAKE UP

Is there any room for improvement to optimize waking up? Yes, and here are some tips:

- Get enough sleep by going to bed early.

- Try to be consistent and wake up at the same time every day. If you are waking up 2 hours later on the weekends, it is a fair sign that you are not getting restorative sleep during the week.

- Open your curtains or turn on your overhead light immediately after waking up so that you can get fast, bright light exposure.

- Take a quick, 5- to 15-minute morning walk. Water your plants, check the bird feeder, play with your dog in the backyard, brush off your car. Do anything that will take you out of the house and into bright daylight.

## WHAT'S NEXT

Making lifestyle changes is one of the fundamental ways in which to address diabetes. This idea isn't new, but the way you establish these new behavioral habits is. In the last four chapters, you have learned about the three critical lifestyle components related to enhancing your circadian rhythm: when you eat, when you exercise, and when you sleep. Now that you know exactly what you need to do and when to do it, you can implement the program and begin to see positive results. As I've said, IF works synergistically with the right foods, the right exercise, and better sleep. Any one of these improvements will add something positive to your overall quality of life, but the three together will yield the most benefits. This program is the best way I know to reverse prediabetes, lower your risk factors for developing diabetes, manage your blood glucose better, and reduce your risk for developing the sinister friends of diabetes.

In the next section, you will learn how to apply these lessons to real life. I have presented a 12-week challenge that you can follow, making incremental changes to ramp you up to optimal circadian code. I hope you will see such great improvement that you'll be convinced to stick with this as your new lifestyle.

The second most important component for improving your blood glucose is to work closely with your doctor as a team. In the next chapter, you will learn how to combine your doctor's advice with what has been presented in this book. Our studies have shown that this is the best way to amplify the common medical practices to get even better results, and this holds true whether you're currently taking medication, or if you've been told you're prediabetic or diabetic, or whether you have been living with diabetes for ten years or more.

Your doctor can help you improve your health if she or he has the right information that accurately relates to how you feel and how your body is changing with this new alignment. In the next chapter, you will learn how to best monitor and assess how you feel day to day, week to week, and month to month. With this information you can compile records that show your good health is progressing as you follow the program. When it comes to diabetes, the proof is literally in your laboratory test scores and daily blood glucose readings.

PART III

# 12 Weeks
# to Reversing Diabetes

## CHAPTER 9

# Managing and Reversing Diabetes Symptoms

Diabetes requires proactive care. As you've learned, living in better alignment with your circadian code can make managing and reversing this disease and its associated symptoms and conditions easier now, as well as going forward. The reason is that when you eat, exercise, and sleep at the right times, you automatically lower your blood glucose levels. And when that happens, all other aspects of your health improve and the symptoms you might be dealing with may lessen.

Yet although these lifestyle changes are powerful medicine, you must still work with your doctor to monitor and improve your health. Diabetes is an insidious disease: it creeps up on you without much warning, making it difficult to detect on your own. Diabetes is like living by a riverbank where the water level is slowly rising; you think that everything is fine and then one day the water washes over the bank and floods your home. When you are prediabetic or even in the early stages of diabetes, you may think that you feel perfectly fine, but you might complain from time to time that you are fatigued or have the occasional aches here and there. Don't ignore those signals: they occur when the river is starting to rise. The only difference between a flood and diabetes is that when the flood subsides and the town is cleaned up, you can rebuild your home and restart your life. But once your blood glucose starts rising year after year, it is not going to go down on its own.

This chapter provides the tools you need to work with your doctor to make the most of every medical visit. Your doctor will be thankful that you have done this work. In fact, showing your doctor that you care enough about your health will give him or her extra incentive to deliver excellent care.

## PREPARING FOR YOUR DOCTOR VISIT

Your doctor can be your best friend on this health journey. But good doctors can do a great job only when they have accurate information about you at their fingertips. To make the most of every visit, including your annual checkup, come prepared. Use a large notebook or binder to collect and arrange your research and bring it with you to every doctor's visit. Then, record what you have learned and keep good records of how you are feeling between visits so that you can determine how you are progressing.

Your binder should include:

YOUR HEALTH HISTORY. Doctors typically ask you to fill out a form annually that lists what health conditions you have experienced in the past year (previous surgeries, eating disorders, unexplained dizziness, etc.). It's hard to remember everything when you aren't feeling great. That's why I recommend thinking about this before your visit and writing down your observations in a notebook.

Your family's health history is also important for your doctor to know; this encompasses diseases and conditions that your blood relatives have had, including your siblings, parents, aunts, and uncles. The information is very important for your own health, as well as the health of your children so that they know what health issues run in their family.

For example, I have a 70-year-old, award-winning colleague who researches the effects of genes and diseases. One day he had emergency bypass surgery. We were shocked at the news, because he was so trim and exceptionally athletic. When he came back to the office, he told us that he had no idea heart disease ran in his family. But during his recovery, his cousin reminded him of an incident that happened when he was a little child. His extended family was visiting from overseas, and he was asked to give up his room for one of his uncles. That night, as his uncle slept in his bed, the uncle died of a massive heart attack. He also found out that there were many other family members who had died from heart disease before the age of 60. Luckily for my colleague, his attention to nutrition and exercise had kept him relatively healthy for more than ten years before he faced a major heart problem, and that also allowed him to have a faster recovery. Now he can share his genetic information with his children and grandchildren, so that they are better prepared.

Talk to your parents, siblings, and other close relatives to find out if any have diabetes and whether they have suffered from any of the health conditions often associated with diabetes, including heart disease, dementia, kidney disease, skin or foot disease, dental diseases, neuropathy or loss of sensation, and certain types of cancer. Check if your mother had gestational diabetes during any pregnancy. Knowing any family history of diabetes or its complications, and sharing that information with your doctor, will help your doctor pay specific attention to potential diabetes complications you may develop in the future and, as a result, he or she will order the relevant lab tests before such symptoms appear.

PRIOR LABORATORY TEST RESULTS. If you have prior test results, bring them to your doctor's visit. This way you can check to see if there is a trend in either a good or a bad direction. In some states, patients can ask their doctor for a copy of previous test results; in others, patients have to pay to see their own lab results. Check with your doctor to determine what records you are entitled to keep for yourself.

MEDICATIONS LIST. Keep a record of which medications you are currently taking and the most current dosages. Your pharmacist should be able to print out this list for you. Include any supplements you are taking, as well as any over-the-counter medicines you take frequently (at least once a week). Make sure to list all medications, even if they are for unrelated problems. For example, some painkillers may produce an abnormal liver function test that would look like a serious liver disease. Go over this list with your doctor at each checkup so you are both aware of any negative interactions between medications.

IMMUNIZATION RECORD. Having diabetes makes you more susceptible to infections and infectious diseases, and if you get a bug, you may suffer more than those without diabetes. A clear example is COVID-19; those with diabetes are at a higher risk for serious COVID-19 complications.[1] Similarly, some diabetes medications, or other meds you may be taking for the sinister friends of diabetes, can make a treatment plan for infectious disease more limited or complicated, which further worsens outcomes. Therefore, it is important to be up to date with available vaccinations.

Adults should be current on the following vaccinations:

- COVID-19 vaccine

- Hepatitis A

- Hepatitis B

- Influenza (the annual flu vaccine)

- Pneumococcal vaccine (pneumonia)

- Shingles vaccine (herpes zoster)

- Tdap (tetanus, diphtheria, pertussis) vaccine and/or booster

RECENT AND UPCOMING LIFE CHANGES. Travel, moving, a new baby, a new job, or any other big-ticket items of life can affect your blood glucose levels. Even happy occasions create new stress, which elevates blood glucose. Also, temporary life changes can cause you to be less diligent about managing your circadian rhythm and overall lifestyle. For example, I once had to travel to a city that is ranked among the top five cities in the United States for adult obesity, diabetes, or high blood pressure. I was staying at a fancy hotel in town. At breakfast, I didn't see any fruit listed on the menu. I asked the concierge where I could buy some, and he told me that I should check three blocks on either side of the hotel. In California, you can get fresh fruit at a 7-Eleven, but even in the fanciest part of this city, I couldn't even find an apple. For lunch we went to a decent restaurant. Again, I skimmed the menu for a low-GI choice, like a salad. The only vegetable on the menu was an avocado appetizer, which was filled with cheese and deep fried. Needless to say, that eating day wasn't great for my blood glucose.

"HOW DO YOU FEEL" CHECKLIST. Use the symptoms listed in the assessment beginning on page 72 as a checklist to assess for doctor's visits. Make a copy of it and keep it in your binder. Every time you go to the doctor, record any symptoms you may be having, especially those that have lasted for at least two months. One way to remember how long you've been dealing with something is to write down the date when the symptom first began. If it goes away in a day or two, it's likely it's nothing to worry about and you can take it off your list.

PROGRESS WITH IF AND OTHER CIRCADIAN ADJUSTMENTS. The progress charts in Chapter 10 are an excellent way to show your doctor what you've learned in this book and what you are implementing. As I've said before, your doctor needs this information because if you've already lowered your blood glucose, that may affect your medication prescription. Better still, your doctor may learn something new. Show the doctor the references in the back of this book to illustrate the research backing up this program.

Your doctor may not know about the most recent circadian rhythm research, although she or he may have heard of IF. If you find that you're feeling much better on IF, share the good news with your doctor. That way, when another person comes to see that doctor, your good experience may lead the doctor to recommend it.

If your doctor is less than receptive to IF, try the following counterargument. Ask the doctor if he or she believes that you should be eating all the time and limiting your opportunities for sleep and exercise. Ask if the doctor thinks any of these disturbances are contributing to your bad health. No doctor will tell you that waking up in the middle of the night and eating a bowl of cereal is a great health strategy. Lastly, remind the doctor that you are going to be seeing him or her every year, reporting on how you're benefiting from the program.

### HOW OFTEN SHOULD I BE GOING TO THE DOCTOR?

Unfortunately, most of us don't go to the doctor as often as we should. This is true for people with or without diabetes; the annual checkup is not a popular pastime. But unless you work with a doctor, you will never know the severity of your health problems.

At minimum, everyone should see a primary care physician annually for a checkup. If you are already being monitored or treated for diabetes, you'll be seeing your doctor at least every year. If you have been living with diabetes for five years or more, you should be seeing your doctor twice a year. The difference hangs on your hemoglobin A1c level: if it is above 7%, then you should see the doctor at least twice a year; if you are below 7, then you can go once a year. Schedule a visit with your doctor after the 12-week program is finished, but if in the past your hemoglobin A1c level has been above 7%, schedule a checkup before you begin. With the new telehealth tools, you can even video-chat with your doctor from the comfort of your home, which cuts out the driving, parking, and waiting time. So, take advantage of these opportunities and meet virtually in your living room to share your diabetes journey.

## LISTEN CAREFULLY FOR THE DIABETES SECRET CODE

Seeing a doctor to talk about diabetes prevention or management is almost like going to an emergency room with a cut on your hand when everyone else in the waiting room is having a heart attack. Your physician may be treating lots of patients who have higher blood glucose levels than yours and other debilitating complications. So, compared to those patients, you may be *doing fine*—but that doesn't mean that you are in perfect health.

If you think back to earlier annual checkups, you may have been confused by what your doctor had told you. For example, the doctor may have reviewed your lab work and told you to pay better attention to your lifestyle—to eat less and move more. Well, that's never bad advice; you've heard it plenty of times from celebrities, friends, and possibly your spouse. You might have thought that your doctor had just joined that chorus and was repeating what's in the ether. What you missed, though, is that those words are actually a code: they mean that you have prediabetes or that your blood pressure and/or cholesterol level has gone up. The truth is, the standard medical practice for addressing prediabetes is *not* to treat the condition with a medication. Instead, that means this lifestyle recommendation is actually a prescription, and it is just as valid as one for medication.

Understanding this language is really important. For example, my friend Sam told me that his doctor has been telling him to eat less and exercise more for years, but it wasn't until he had to talk to his doctor about getting a COVID test that he learned he was prediabetic. This was a gigantic and worrisome surprise, especially because Sam knew that people with diabetes had a much more difficult time with the coronavirus. Now Sam is taking those recommendations more seriously.

## TELL YOUR DOCTOR EXACTLY HOW YOU FEEL

How you *feel* is an important aspect of your diabetes management plan. Yet many people don't discuss their symptoms or their discomfort with their doctor. Some may believe that the aches and pains common among their friends are normal effects of aging, but that is not true. If you're feeling pain anywhere, if you're having more dental issues than in the past, or even if you are tired all the time, those can be early signs of diabetes. Your doctor needs to know how you are feeling so as to have a better assessment of your health.

While you will feel better following the recommendations outlined in Part II, know that those changes will not happen overnight. You may still have symptoms, and for the first week or two you might develop new ones as your body adjusts to your different schedule. Keep taking your medication and give yourself time to adjust. Next week will be better.

Some symptoms will resolve within four to six weeks on the program, like sleep quality and fatigue. Some might take longer. For example, reducing your cholesterol or improving your HDL cholesterol might take six months to a year. In our studies, changes to blood sugar and weight loss may take between 6 and 12 weeks. Blurred vision will not improve with this program: get an eye exam with full dilation from an optometrist or ophthalmologist once a year.

In the meantime, review the health assessment on page 72 that lists all of the possible symptoms again. The most common diabetes symptoms include (arranged alphabetically):

- Blurred vision

- Extreme hunger

- Fatigue

- Frequent infections, such as gums or skin infections and vaginal infections

- Frequent urination

- Increased thirst

- Irritability

- Slow-healing sores

- Unexplained weight loss

**GO TO THE DENTIST**

Diabetes and dental disease often occur together. Diabetes can weaken connective tissues, including the part of the mouth that holds a tooth to the jawbone, and teeth can become loose. A second issues is microvascular disease. With diabetes, the blood circulation to the teeth can be altered, which can also weaken them.

Lastly, there can be tooth decay because of the side effects of diabetes. You should be seeing a dentist regularly, but you may want to make an additional trip if you notice anything unusual.

And remember, just because you have a clean bill of health from the dentist does not mean that you're not prediabetic. Don't take your good news from your dentist as your having passed the diabetes test.

## UNDERSTANDING YOUR LAB RESULTS

Frequent testing is the best way to make sure you are progressing. No matter what kind of diabetes risk you may have, get your fasting blood glucose and a few others (oral glucose tolerance/postprandial glucose, random test, hemoglobin A1c, and anemia) tested at least once a year. I mentioned these tests in Chapter 1; your doctor uses them to make an initial diagnosis. Now I want you to continue taking these tests, year after year, to chart your progress. Some of these tests you will even be able to do at home.

Most people go to their annual checkup, get a lab order for blood work, and then get their labs done. If the results come back outside the normal range, your doctor may call you with some advice or a prescription. A more proactive approach is to turn the visit around. As soon as you get a date for your checkup, ask your doctor for a lab test order. This way you can do your blood work ahead of time and then spend the office visit talking about the results.

Ask your doctor to provide you with your numbers, even if the response is *"Don't worry, everything is normal/fine."* For example, if you have gotten your HbA1c tested every year for three years and it has always been within the healthy range (<5.6%), yet it has risen from 5.1 to 5.3 to 5.5%, you can clearly see an upward trend. If you don't change your current lifestyle, you may become prediabetic next year, when it crosses the 5.6 threshold. And if you don't like the number you heard, but your doctor doesn't believe that the number is bad enough to warrant a more serious conversation, know that just by following this program the trend will move in the right direction.

Most doctors may order only the standard tests. I suggest you request all of the following tests. Some may be covered by your insurance and some may not be. Check how much they will cost both with and without insurance coverage and, depending on your financial situation, get as many tests as possible. You can get your standard blood work done before you start the program, then again after 12 weeks. The basic tests you should have are the fasting blood glucose, hemoglobin A1c, blood pressure, cholesterol, and triglyceride lab tests. Your family health history will also help you determine if you need other specific tests.

## GROUP 1: BLOOD GLUCOSE ASSESSMENTS

FASTING BLOOD GLUCOSE. This is the only standard test to determine if you are diabetic, and it is the one you have to take in the morning on an empty stomach. It offers a snapshot of your blood glucose only for that day. Again, pay close attention to your numbers, even if they are on the border of the prediabetic range. If you have been told that you are in the prediabetes stage, then you can completely reverse the disease and get your blood sugar back within the normal range. If you're in the early stages of diabetes, you can better manage the disease and lower your numbers. And if you're severely diabetic, and if you're paying attention, then you can reduce the collateral damage that can be done to your heart, kidneys, and other organs. You can do this test in the doctor's office or at home.

**Normal** = less than 100 mg/dL

**Prediabetes** = 100–125 mg/dL

**Diabetes** = >126–170 mg/dL

**Severe diabetes** = >170 mg/dL

HEMOGLOBIN A1C. This test shows your history of blood glucose for the last three months. Even if your fasting blood glucose is less than 100 mg/dL, ask your doctor to do a hemoglobin A1c because your fasting blood glucose does not take into account how high your blood sugar is throughout the day. You can do this test in the doctor's office.

**Normal** = <5.6%

**Prediabetes** = 5.7–6.4%

**Diabetes** = >6.5%

ORAL GLUCOSE TOLERANCE /POSTPRANDIAL GLUCOSE. This test will let you know how your body reacts to food. If you scored 5 or more on the diabetes risk factors in Chapter 1, or your fasting blood glucose result is in the prediabetes range, ask your doctor to order this test. You can do this test in the doctor's office or with a finger prick test at home. You will wait for two hours after drinking a standard sugary drink with 75 grams of glucose. If your blood glucose level remains at 200 mg/dL or higher, then you have diabetes. At home, you can test yourself two hours after any standard-size meal; if your blood sugar remains above 200 mg/dL, you are diabetic. For pregnant women, if this number remains at 140 mg/dL or higher, then you have gestational diabetes.

ANEMIA. Symptoms of anemia include fatigue, light-headedness, dizziness, or a rapid heartbeat, which overlaps with some symptoms of diabetes. Anemia can affect your hemoglobin A1c result and may yield an unusually low or high number that does not accurately report your blood glucose history. If your hemoglobin A1c numbers are off, your doctor may recommend this test or other tests that determine the quality of your blood cells. A normal reading varies based on your sex and age, and if you are pregnant. A hemoglobin concentration reading of 7.0 to 11 g/dL is considered moderate anemia, and 7.0 g/dL or less is considered severe anemia. You can do this test in the doctor's office.

## GROUP 2: COMPLICATIONS OF DIABETES ASSESSMENTS

BLOOD PRESSURE, SYSTOLIC AND DIASTOLIC. These are standard tests performed at every annual checkup. High or low blood pressure cannot tell you if you have diabetes, but it can tell you if you are at risk of developing heart diseases. Diabetes can make you prone to high blood pressure, and diabetes with high blood pressure can increase your risk for heart disease. You can do this test in the doctor's office or at home.

**Normal** = 90–120 systolic, 60–80 diastolic

**Pre-high blood pressure** = 120–140 systolic, 80–90 diastolic

**High blood pressure** = >140 systolic, >90 diastolic

CHOLESTEROL SCREENS: BLOOD CHOLESTEROL, TOTAL CHOLESTEROL, AND LDL AND HDL CHOLESTEROL. These are standard tests performed at every annual checkup. High cholesterol cannot tell you if you have diabetes, but just like high blood pressure, it can tell you if you are at high risk for heart disease or stroke. You can do this test in the doctor's office.

**Total cholesterol:** One test that includes LDL, HDL, and others. It is more important to pay attention to both LDL and HDL numbers.

**LDL (or L for lousy or bad) cholesterol:**

Normal = <100 mg/dL with no history of heart disease, <70 mg/dL with history of heart disease

**HDL (or H for healthy or good) cholesterol:**

Normal = >60 mg/dL

Borderline = 40–60 mg/dL

Too low = <40 mg/dL

BLOOD TRIGLYCERIDE. This is a standard test performed at every annual checkup. Blood triglyceride levels cannot tell you if you have diabetes, but in combination with diabetes and bad cholesterol, they can tell you if you have a higher chance of heart disease. You can do this test in the doctor's office.

**Normal** = <100 mg/dL

LIVER FUNCTION (AST, ALT). If you are overweight or obese, or prediabetic, you can ask for a liver function test, which will show whether your liver is working fine or if there are excess fat deposits that make it work less effectively. A bad liver test can be a signal that you are likely to progress to more severe diabetes in the future. You can do this test in the doctor's office.

**Normal AST** = 5–50 units/Liter of blood

**Normal ALT** = 7–56 units/Liter of blood

KIDNEY FUNCTION. There are many kidney function tests, including Glomerular Filtration Rate, Serum Creatinine, and Urinary Albumin-to-Creatine Ratio. Kidney function tests are only performed when you know there is a family history of kidney disease, or if you are frequently going to the bathroom two or three times during the hours when you should be sleeping. You should also check for the presence of ketones in urine. Ketones are a by-product of the breakdown of muscle and fat. Dangerously high levels happen when there's not enough available insulin in your system, not from following a ketogenic diet. Usually, ketones are undetectable in urine, so any amount of detectable ketone in the urine is a sign of diabetes.

**Blood Urea Nitrogen (BUN):** Normal = 7–20 mg/dL

**Serum Creatinine:** Normal = 0.84–1.21 mg/dL

**Albumin Urea Test (urine test):**

Normal = <30 mg/dL

Potential kidney damage = 30–300 mg/dL

Severe kidney damage = >300 mg

VITAMIN B$_{12}$. If you're already taking the diabetes medication metformin (Glucophage, Riomet, Glumetza, Glucophage XR, or Fortamet), you need to check your vitamin B$_{12}$ levels. One of the side effects of metformin is that it lowers your ability to absorb vitamin B$_{12}$, which can make you feel weak and depressed, and can contribute to numbness in toes (peripheral neuropathy).

**Normal** = 180–914 ng/L (nanogram/liter of blood)

THYROID (TSH). If you have Type 1 diabetes, feel lethargic, or have unexplained weight gain, ask your doctor to test your thyroid gland. Women over 40 years of age who are premenopausal or menopausal typically have less thyroid function. An overactive or underactive thyroid cannot tell if you have diabetes, but it can explain a rapid weight gain or weight loss, or feelings of anxiety or lethargy. You can do this test in the doctor's office. If you are outside of the normal range your doctor will recommend further testing.

COMPREHENSIVE FOOT EXAM. Your doctor can check your feet for any numbness or lack of sensation, which are symptoms of severe diabetes. If your doctor tells you that you have a concerning level of numbness, consider wearing comfortable shoes like sneakers all the time, and check your feet every day for cuts, bruises, or skin abnormalities.

## RULES FOR REGULAR TESTING

Keep the following in mind before you get your blood tests:

- Always go for your blood work at the same time of day, preferably in the morning (before 10 a.m.) and on an empty stomach. If you take your blood tests before 10:00 a.m., then it's likely that your overnight fast is about the same length as usual. If you take the tests after 10:00 or 11:00 a.m., then you might have fasted more than 14 to 16 hours, which can change the test results. Do not drink anything besides water before your blood test.

- Make sure you can maintain your normal lifestyle and schedule for at least three days prior to the tests. Try to get a good night's sleep and limit your consumption of fatty foods or excess alcohol. Fatty, fried foods can affect the blood work for more than a day, while the effect of having excess carbs dissipates within 12 hours. If you do night shift work, try to get your tests done on an off day when you can fast ahead of time for at least 10 hours.

- Don't test immediately after having a fever, cold, flu, or infection. The illness itself or the medication to treat it can affect your lab results.

## MAYA TOOK HER NUMBERS SERIOUSLY AND REVERSED PREDIABETES

Maya is in her mid-30s, working as a sales manager at a multinational company. She typically travels on business several times a year. Last year, after her annual checkup, her doctor told her everything was fine, but when Maya was about to leave the appointment, the doctor suggested that Maya "just watch your diet and do some exercise." Maya thought the comment was strange, as she hadn't gained any weight in the past five years, and during physicals in those years her doctor never mentioned that she needed to diet.

When she got home, she dug up her lab results from the last four years and compared them with the numbers on the sheet her doctor had just given her. Being in sales, she was quick to spot the trends. Her fasting blood sugar had been creeping up over the last four years from 83 to 89, 96, 101, and now 116 mg/dL. Similarly, her HbA1c for the same period was 4.7, 4.9, 5.2, 5.4, and 5.9%. Even though her doctor didn't use the words "you're prediabetic," Maya knew what the results meant: her mother has Type 2 diabetes. Maya's blood cholesterol was also creeping up and was now at 229 mg/dL (considered borderline high).

Maya wanted to try IF to reverse her prediabetes. She considered her lifestyle when she set up her eating window, knowing her business travel and typical late-night dinners with clients would affect her timing, so she selected a 10-hour eating window that stretched from 11:00 a.m. to 9:00 p.m. She planned to skip the breakfast meal and instead have brunch around 11:00 a.m., one or two healthy snacks in the afternoon, and her business dinner starting at 7:00 p.m. She swapped her 8:30 a.m. morning latte for a black coffee with no sugar or cream. She was doing what I call the "black coffee IF," which is okay because while it's not the perfect way to do IF, it is better than not doing IF at all.

Maya also bought a blood glucose monitor to check her morning fasting blood glucose once every week. After 12 weeks her morning fasting blood glucose had come down to between 101 and 110 mg/dL. She also felt sharper during the day and had better sleep at night, including on her travel days (which was a pleasant bonus surprise for her). She noticed that her menstrual cycle was more regular now. She had always thought traveling once a month might have been the reason for her irregular periods, but the new IF lifestyle restored her peace of mind about her reproductive health.

She continued this lifestyle, and after six months of IF, when Maya got her labs done again, her prediabetes was gone. Her fasting glucose stood at 95 mg/dL, her HbA1c was at 5.4%, and her cholesterol had come down to 196 mg/dL. All these numbers were technically healthy. But Maya knows that she has to maintain this lifestyle if she wants to continue to enjoy good health.

## ASSESS YOUR MEDICATIONS

Your doctor will determine if you need to start taking medication to control diabetes, or whether you can make a change to the medications you are already taking. This is an important decision to make with your doctor. We have been trained to feel that getting a prescription from a doctor is a sign of success, and that our symptoms or condition will magically disappear as a result. While that may be true for some health issues, it isn't true for diabetes. Yes, you may feel better when your blood sugar is controlled with medication. However, taking the medication is only one small part of a diabetes management program. Any prescription is not a free pass to revert to old ways that may have caused your condition in the first place.

The biggest contributor to improvement is paying attention to your lifestyle by optimizing your circadian rhythm. Remember, if you don't correct your lifestyle, then that first diabetes pill can become two pills in a year, and three or four pills in two to three years. Worse, if you rely solely on medication to control your blood glucose, over time your blood glucose levels can worsen. That's why you'll often hear that someone who has diabetes has to increase the dose over time. My goal is for you to take less medication over time, not more.

One reason I feel strongly about making these lifestyle interventions is that it takes a medicine cabinet to manage diabetes, and many of those medications can produce adverse side effects that range from general weakness to stomach issues, pain, and other symptoms. Generally, the higher the dose of the medication, the higher the risk of adverse effects; then, to take care of these side effects, you may have to take additional drugs. So, it is not surprising that the average person living with a diagnosis of Type 2 diabetes for five years or more takes *six* or more prescription medications.[2] What's more, the more meds you have to take, the more likely it will be that you will forget to take them on time or every day.

Also, be aware that certain diabetes medications can cause severe hypoglycemia when combined with IF. If you are already taking diabetes medications and find that you feel dizzy when you start IF, stop the program and talk to your doctor. Your doctor may adjust your medication before you restart a 10- or 12-hour eating regimen.

If you are on blood pressure medications or cholesterol medication, discuss IF with your doctor before you start the program. You may not need to reduce the dosage before you start IF, but you may want to get yourself checked every three months after implementing IF, to adjust all drug dosage, or even get off some medications.

## DIFFERENT TYPES OF DIABETES MEDICATIONS, WHAT THEY DO (MODE OF ACTION), AND THEIR TYPICAL COMPLICATIONS

| Type of Drug | Trade Names (US) | Comparative Cost | Oral or Injection | Effective for Glucose Control | Risk for Developing Hypoglycemia |
|---|---|---|---|---|---|
| Metformin | Fortamet, Glucophage XR, Glumetza, Riomet | Low | Oral | High | No |
| SGLT2 inhibitors | Jardiance, Farxiga, Invokana | High | Oral | Intermediate | No |
| GLP1-RAs | Victoza, Saxenda, Adlyxin, Ozempic, Rybelsus, Trulicity, Byetta, Bydureon | High | Oral or injection | High | No |
| DPP-4 inhibitors | Januvia, Onglyza, Tradjenta, Nesina, Vipidia | High | Oral | Intermediate | No |
| Thiazolidinediones | Actos, Avandia | Low | Oral | High | No |
| Sulfonylureas (2nd generation) | Glucotrol, Diamicron, Gliben-J, Daonil, DiaBeta, Euglucon, Glurenorm | Low | Oral | High | Yes |
| Insulin | Lantus, Humalog, Levemir, NovoLog, Apidra, Tresiba | Medium-high | Injection or inhaled | Highest | Yes |

Different types of diabetes medications and their efficacy to reduce blood glucose and potential side effects. Only some of the trade names are shown. Several diabetes medications (not shown here) also contain a combination of metformin and another drug and are marketed under different trade names. Within the same class of drugs, depending on dose or chemical formula, some may have adverse effects, whereas others may not. Your doctor may take into account your kidney function and risk for future kidney diseases when prescribing specific diabetes medications and their dosage.

| Type of Drug | Weight Change | Arterial Plaque Buildup | Heart Failure | Other Potential Risks/ Side Effects |
|---|---|---|---|---|
| Metformin | Neutral | Potential benefit | Neutral | Upset stomach, vitamin $B_{12}$ deficiency |
| SGLT2 inhibitors | Weight Loss | Benefit | Benefit | Bone fracture, amputation, urinary tract infection, low blood pressure, increased LDL cholesterol |
| GLP1-RAs | Weight Loss | Mostly neutral | Neutral | Upset stomach, pancreas inflammation, thyroid cancer |
| DPP-4 inhibitors | Neutral | Neutral | Some risk from certain drugs | Pancreas inflammation, joint pain |
| Thiazolidinediones | Weight Gain | Some drugs may benefit | Increased risk | Heart failure (for some drugs), fluid retention, bone fractures, bladder cancer, increased LDL cholesterol |
| Sulfonylureas (2nd generation) | Weight Gain | Neutral | Neutral | Feeling low energy (due to potential hypoglycemia at night), heart failure based on first-generation drugs |
| Insulin | Weight Gain | Neutral | Neutral | Injection site reaction, hypoglycemia |

## MANAGING DIABETES WITH OPTIMAL TIMING OF MEDICATION

One way to reduce your dependence on medication is to make sure you are taking your prescriptions at the right time of day. Just like our bodily functions have circadian rhythms, the body responds to certain drugs better at specific times. Aligning with that "right time" to take the meds can potentially reduce adverse side effects and make the drugs more effective, even to the point where you may be able to take a lower dose.

Diabetes medications typically reduce blood glucose after a meal. That's why the right time for taking most medications is just before or immediately after breakfast, lunch, or dinner. One class of drugs called sulfonylureas can reduce your fasting blood sugar level irrespective of your meal. If those medications are taken in the evening, then they are more likely to cause more harm by further reducing your blood sugar level to dangerously low levels. So, those are the only drugs that should always be taken in the morning. For all the other medications, just follow what your physician tells you to do. Certain types of diabetes medications (SGLT2 inhibitors) at a low dose are more effective at bedtime compared with morning. However, these medications may cause you to wake up to use the bathroom in the middle of the night. If you don't mind waking up once during the night to use the bathroom, you can try taking these specific diabetes medications in the evening. Insulin is always taken before eating.

People take different types of supplements or vitamins. For example, doctors often tell patients on metformin to take vitamin $B_{12}$ at the same time. And many diabetes patients have joint problems so they add medications to treat that joint pain. If you have arthritis or joint pain, although the pain is worse in the morning, take the pain medication at bedtime. A slow-release formulation of the pain med at bedtime works better to reduce arthritis pain in the morning.[3,4]

A sinister friend of diabetes is hypertension, or high blood pressure. Irrespective of what type of blood pressure medication you might be on, taking the medication at bedtime is always better than taking it in the morning. Some studies have shown that evening statins are better, and other studies have shown better results for morning statins. The difference might have to do with dosage or type of statin. A recent study on blood pressure medication timing and outcome showed that blood pressure meds, if taken at bedtime, have better outcomes than the same medications taken in the morning or after breakfast.[5]

## BE HONEST WITH YOUR DOCTOR REGARDING COMPLIANCE

If you are not regularly taking your medications, be honest with your doctor. Otherwise, your doctor may prescribe more powerful medications, thinking that the one you are taking isn't working if your blood glucose levels are moving in the wrong direction.

As I mentioned, some medications have unpleasant side effects. Some diabetes medications can cause upset stomach, some can cause nightly hypoglycemia, some can affect kidney function and cause frequent urination, some can induce a urinary tract infection. If you are not taking your medication because it is causing other problems, discuss this situation with your doctor. The doctor may prescribe a lower dose or an alternate medication, or give you different instructions for when to take your meds so that you can tolerate them better.

## MONITOR YOUR HEALTH WITH THE RIGHT TOOLS

Investing in some basic tools will make managing your diabetes infinitely easier. Many of these tools will be useful for everyone in your family—even those without diabetes.

BODY WEIGHT SCALE. A simple bathroom scale is fine, but if you want to be fancy, get one with a Wi-Fi connection that can automatically transmit your weight to a log kept on your smartphone. Weighing yourself once a week is sufficient—you don't have to weigh every day—but try to weigh yourself at the same time each week. Try to take your weight in the morning after a bowel movement and before eating your breakfast. Your weight can vary by up to 2 pounds during the day, depending on whether you have just eaten a large meal or whether you have some fluid retention.

MEASURING TAPE. One of the measurements of risk for diabetes and heart disease is belly fat, or the waist-to-hip ratio. The easiest way to track this is to take an accurate measurement of your waist once a month. If your waist is more than 40 inches (for men) and 35 inches (for women), talk to your doctor to set a goal for losing weight. Asian men and women are at higher risk and need to further reduce their waistline: $35^1/_2$ inches for men and $31^1/_2$ inches for women. Even if you don't lose too much weight, losing a few pounds from your belly goes a long way toward improving your diabetes situation and reducing your risk for heart disease. We have found that following a 10-hour IF for 12 weeks can lead to a clinically significant reduction in waist circumference.[6]

BLOOD GLUCOSE MONITOR. A simple blood sugar monitor uses finger pricks. Your blood glucose reacts with a chemical on a piece of paper, and the resulting reaction is read by the glucose meter. Many of these monitors now have a Wi-Fi connection to automatically transfer the results to your smartphone or computer. Most of them are covered by insurance and even without insurance, they are considered a tax-deductible medical expense in the United States. You will need a blood glucose monitor for the 12-week challenge outlined in Chapter 10.

Your morning fasting blood glucose can vary from day to day. If you are diabetic, the number may fluctuate as much as 10 to 30 points between days. But if it goes up by more than 30 points relative to the previous day or relative to your last seven-day average, then try to remember what you did differently on the previous day. If you ate a meal too late, did not sleep well, had a change in medication, didn't exercise, or felt sick, your blood glucose can be quite different.

If you are prediabetic, take a fasting blood glucose reading once or twice a month. If you are diabetic, take the reading once or twice a week. If you are severely diabetic or are on insulin therapy, do it every day. No matter how often you take the reading, do it in the morning, immediately after you wake up. Then, take a bedtime blood glucose reading. If you eat your last meal more than 3 hours before bedtime, your blood glucose before bed should be similar to or slightly above your morning fasting glucose level.

If your doctor has recently told you for the first time that you are diabetic, take a fasting blood glucose reading every week. For two to three days each week, take a blood glucose reading before breakfast (i.e., 1 to 2 hours after waking up), lunch, and dinner and then repeat the readings 1 hour after breakfast, lunch, and dinner. If your lunch is 4 or 5 hours after breakfast and dinner is 4 or 5 hours after lunch, your before-meal readings should be similar to your morning fasting glucose (unless you snack in between).

The reading after a meal is mostly determined by the type of food you eat. If you have food rich in carbohydrates, and specifically from sugary or starchy food, then your after-meal blood glucose can spike as high as 160, 180, or even more than 200 mg/dL. But if it shoots up to 300 mg/dL or higher after any one meal, talk to your doctor, because a reading this high means that you may be hyperglycemic and might pass out in the future, even if you feel fine now. This condition may improve with IF that is combined with better food choices, as outlined in Chapter 6.

During IF, if you wake up in the middle of the night feeling too hungry or feeling dizzy from hypoglycemia, and you can take a blood glucose reading before reaching out for some sugary drinks to manage your hypoglycemia, take that glucose reading. If it is unusually low (<70 mg/dL), then make a note of it, take the recovery drink, and in the morning let your doctor know about this. If this pattern repeats within a week or two, try to go back to a 12-hour IF eating window and let your doctor know so your diabetes medications can be adjusted. Your doctor will let you know when you can try the 10-hour eating window again.

CONTINUOUS GLUCOSE MONITOR (CGM). This is a wearable device with a small filament that is inserted under the skin on the belly or on the arm. Once inserted, the CGM takes a glucose reading every 5 or 15 minutes. The device itself is a small disc that attaches to your belly or arm with a temporary glue. Each CGM can be worn for up to two weeks, during which time you can shower, swim, do physical activity, and sleep with it on.

There are three types of CGM monitors. The first is from Abbott called FreeStyle Libre, which is the least expensive, and is only for Type 2 diabetes. The Dexcom G6 CGM and the Medtronic Guardian Connect CGM are both good for Type 1 diabetes. Depending on which CGM you are wearing, the reading can be sent straight to your smartphone. Sometimes you may have to swipe your smartphone against the CGM to get the latest number. The reading will let you know whether you are in a safe range or if you are approaching hypoglycemia or hyperglycemia. Some models also tell you which way you are trending over a period of time—whether your blood sugar is going down, going up, or staying steady.

A CGM is much better than the finger-prick glucose monitor because it continues to test you at night. We aren't exactly sure why nightly blood glucose fluctuates. Although you might think that if you don't eat in the middle of your sleep, your blood glucose remains low and flat, this is not always true. Some people show nightly rises in blood glucose and some show a sharp rise in the morning, even before waking up. These glucose fluctuations can be reduced and stabilized to within a healthy range for many individuals who do IF,[7] as long as they are aware of them.

The CGM also helps you learn how your blood glucose changes after a night of disturbed sleep. For instance, you may see more fluctuation in nightly glucose and a modest increase in glucose on the following day. CGM can also pick up nighttime hypoglycemia before you have any symptoms. The CGMs that are recommended for people with Type 1 diabetes are more reliable in detecting dangerously low glucose or hypoglycemia that can happen in your sleep, or even during the daytime.

There are studies showing that people who use glucose monitors do much better in controlling their blood glucose.[8] A CGM can show you results after every meal, so you can see how high your blood glucose goes and how long it stays above the safe level. As you adjust your diet to include more high-fiber and low-GI foods, you will also notice how the glucose rise may be blunted. By seeing these responses meal after meal, you can choose the foods that do not raise your blood glucose dangerously high. You will be surprised to find that many store-bought, packaged foods that claim to be healthy will, in fact, raise your blood glucose to a dangerous level. At the same time, you may learn that certain snacks, such as peanuts, edamame, and so on, do not raise your blood glucose too much. My study participants have told me that when they eat roasted in-shell peanuts as a snack, their blood glucose barely rises.

A CGM can also help you see how exercise affects your blood glucose in real time. A brisk walk outside or on a treadmill, or on an elliptical or exercise bike, for 10 to 15 minutes before or after a meal will help to keep your blood glucose in check. You may notice a smaller rise and a sharper fall in blood glucose depending on when and how much you exercise before or after a meal. This will help you figure out what type of exercise you can do to optimally reduce your blood glucose. You can also wear a CGM during strenuous exercise; spinning, high-intensity interval training, running, weight training, and the like and see how your blood glucose changes. If your blood glucose goes up too high, consider reducing your exercise intensity. The great thing is that you don't have to remember to do the test because the CGM is doing it all the time. And it's not painful. Having a CGM and taking note of every meal you eat can be a powerful approach to learning about how your own body reacts to different foods at different times of the day. And, you don't have to write down the numbers because you can always look at your history on your smartphone.

If you forget your medicine, you may also see a general rise in your blood sugar—both fasting and postprandial blood glucose may rise; these are two important reminders to take your medication. Lastly, stress can raise your blood glucose level, and you may notice it on your CGM. It can act as a good reminder to incorporate relaxing activities into your daily routine, such as breathing exercises, meditation, and reading.

If you decide to use a CGM, also have a finger prick glucose reader handy. The CGM readings can make you more anxious about your blood glucose until you master using the data. For example, after a meal, the CGM reading is slightly delayed by 15 to 30 minutes relative to your blood glucose reading from a finger prick test. Also, some of the CGMs can occasionally give a reading that is 10 to 20 points higher or lower than the finger prick reading. Some brands of CGMs also misrepresent your fasting blood glucose during sleep, particularly if the sensor is pressed against the mattress or your partner, showing that your blood sugar is too low, while in essence your blood sugar may not be that low.

Unlike a blood glucose monitor that anyone can purchase in the United States, as of 2021, you need a prescription to buy a CGM. Check with your health insurance company to see if it is covered. If you are prediabetic or early-stage diabetic with an HbA1c of less than 7.0%, it is unlikely that your doctor would prescribe a CGM. There are some CGMs that cost less than others, and even the least expensive ones can cost up to $200 per month without insurance. But if your insurance company approves it, that approval will be for three months or up to a year. If your HbA1c is more than 7%, and if your insurance company approves it, then it's better to wear the CGM as frequently as you can. But at minimum, wearing one once every three months for fourteen days will give you a good idea where you are with your blood sugar levels. I recommend that on the 12-week IF program, it would be the most valuable to wear one for the first two weeks and then during the last two weeks.

MEDICINE REMINDER. Most diabetics take more than one medication to manage their blood glucose and associated health conditions. In addition to these, your doctor may prescribe certain vitamins, minerals, and supplements. A weekly pill organizer is an easy tool to make sure that you take medication regularly. You might also use a pill reminder app to signal when it's time to take your meds.

## A CONTINUOUS GLUCOSE MONITOR

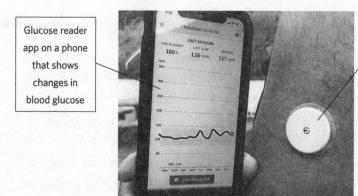

Glucose reader app on a phone that shows changes in blood glucose

Continuous glucose monitor attached to the arm

## HOW THE CGM REPORTS A GLUCOSE READING

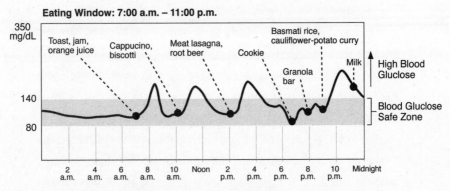

**Eating Window: 7:00 a.m. – 11:00 p.m.**

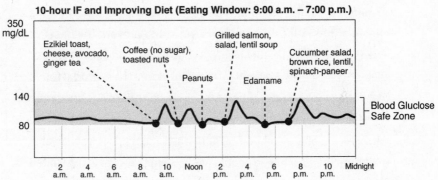

**10-hour IF and Improving Diet (Eating Window: 9:00 a.m. – 7:00 p.m.)**

MEDITERRANEAN DIET COOKBOOK. Almost all cookbooks are written for people without obesity, diabetes, or heart diseases. Most of them do not provide the calorie count or nutrition content for the recipes. However, many cookbooks advocate the Mediterranean diet, like *The Mediterranean Method* by Steven Masley, MD. This cookbook contains that nutritional information, as well as plenty of healthy recipes using fruits, vegetables, fish, and meat. Additionally, you will always find something you can cook by consulting the shopping list beginning on page 142.

### PARTICIPATE IN A CLINICAL STUDY FOR DIABETES MANAGEMENT

Your participation in a clinical study can be fulfilling as you will improve the health of millions of other people. Check ClinicalTrials

.gov for studies being done near you. Search for "diabetes," "weight management," "heart condition," "exercise program," "foot care," and more. If you are part of an ethnic minority, it is even more important that you participate in such studies. Some of the studies may require a specific time commitment. But you will get more care, more medical attention, and more safety monitoring than your current health care or insurance company can provide.

For example, one well-known study tracking diabetes called the Diabetes Prevention Program (DPP), involved 3,234 participants who were at high risk for developing diabetes and it was held at 27 different clinical centers. The participants were tested on the effects of better lifestyle and medications to prevent the onset of Type 2 diabetes (NIDDK.NIH.gov/About-NIDDK/Research-Areas/Diabetes/Diabetes-Prevention-Program-dpp). This study found that reducing body weight by 5% or more and adding moderate physical activity for 150 minutes a week were effective in preventing Type 2 diabetes among 58% of participants. It is conceivable that more than 32 million people will prevent diabetes in the United States alone by following the results of this DPP. That means that every one of those participants contributed to improving the health of at least 10,000 people, or the population of a small town.

Similarly, our own study of 10-hour IF spawned many other studies and initiated a trend in IF. In the last six years, at least 8 million people worldwide have adopted some forms of IF. In other words, each of our early adopters of TRE/IF has influenced the health of at least a million people.

## WHAT'S NEXT

It's time to put everything you've learned together. In the next chapter, I show you how to take the 12-week IF challenge so you can see how you can improve your health.

## CHAPTER 10

# The 12-Week Challenge

The goal of the 12-week challenge is to get all three aspects of your circadian code—eating, exercise, and sleeping—into optimal alignment. This challenge is designed to incorporate both the small and big changes necessary, so that you can adopt and sustain IF for the rest of your life. The overwhelming consensus from our research is that once people adopt a 10-hour Intermittent Fasting window, everything else becomes easy to incorporate. As I like to say, good habits beget more good habits.

The challenge is designed to help you make incremental changes instead of bombarding you with multiple large changes all at once. It is also designed to last for 12 weeks because that is the time necessary to both create new habits and track real progress. I have outlined the program to feature biweekly changes. Stick as best as you can to the schedule. If you are up to a greater challenge, you can always incorporate the exercise or sleep strategies for the upcoming two weeks earlier. When it comes to exercise and sleep, more is always better.

We have also found that food-choice compliance is the most difficult aspect of the challenge. My advice is to get your family on board with this new eating plan as quickly as possible. The more people in your household that you can convert to a low-GI Mediterranean diet, the easier it will be to stick with it. Remember, we're not counting a single calorie: we are focusing on making better choices. Before long, your whole family will see how many new delicious food options are available and easy to prepare.

Let's get started!

## SET YOURSELF UP FOR SUCCESS

The following items will make it easier to succeed in the challenge because they can enhance your optimization of IF, sleep, and exercise.

- **Notebook.** You can use the same notebook in which you are keeping your medical history; that way you can show your progress to your doctor. During the challenge, you will keep detailed records to log your food, fasting time, sleep time, and so on. You can also use your smartphone or the myCircadianClock app.

- **Earplugs, nose strips, and an eye mask.** These can assist you in getting a good night's sleep at home or when you travel. If you are a frequent traveler, you may also want a comfortable neck pillow for in-flight naps.

- **Sneakers/exercise shoes.** Purchase comfortable walking shoes with a good insole. If you have lost sensation in your leg, it is even more important to make sure you wear protective shoes all the time to avoid getting injured and infected. If you are overweight or obese and want to start brisk walking or weight training, consult a trainer to purchase braces (e.g., knee braces) to prevent sore or sprained joints.

- **Refillable water bottle.** These are a great way to see how much water you have consumed, which is difficult to track if you are pouring yourself only a glass a couple of times a day.

- **Blood glucose monitor.** These are available at any drugstore. See if your doctor can also prescribe a continuous glucose monitor; though not essential, it is nice to have.

- **Home blood pressure monitor.** These are available at any drugstore and are simple to use.

## SET YOUR PERSONAL GOALS

Personal goals are just that—they work for you, and you alone. You know how you are living and what your current state of health is. And you know what is coming up for you in the near future. For now, let's set the goals just for this 12-week challenge.

Your goals can be influenced by what your doctor has told you about your blood glucose numbers. The numbers don't lie and monitoring them is the best way to determine if you are succeeding. And as you learned in Chapter 1, lowering your blood glucose is even more important than weight loss. So, let's begin by writing down your top three goals. They can be specifically about your mental or physical health. Here are some ideas you can work with.

*If you have prediabetes with HbA1c between 5.6 and 6.5% or a fasting blood glucose between 100 and 125 mg/dL:

1.  Reverse my HbA1c to within healthy range
2.  Reduce my risk for metabolic syndrome
3.  Improve physical fitness by walking at least 5,000 steps a day and doing some stretching and strength exercises

*If you are living with Type 2 diabetes and take only one diabetes medication:

1.  Reduce my HbA1c by 0.5%
2.  Reduce my risk for metabolic syndrome
3.  Improve physical fitness by walking at least 5,000 steps a day and doing some stretching and strength exercises

*If you are living with diabetes and take two or more diabetes medications:

1.  Reduce my HbA1c by 0.5%
2.  Reduce my diabetes medication dosage
3.  Reduce my symptoms for diabetes and its complications

Personal Goal #1: _____

Personal Goal #2: _____

Personal Goal #3: _____

## SET YOUR WEIGHT AND HEALTH GOALS

Use the chart in Chapter 1 to determine how much weight you need to lose. Find your target weight for the challenge by assuming that you will lose an average of 1 pound a week. If you are significantly overweight, you may lose more. As you lose weight, your waistline will likely decrease; it's a good goal for both men and women to lose 1 inch around the waist or go down 1 pant size. The CDC recommends that you use a tape measure, measuring your waist around your belly button.[1]

Record your current measurements and goals:

Height: _____

Beginning Weight: _____

Target Weight: _____

Beginning Waist Circumference: _____

Target Waist Circumference: _____

Current Morning Fasting Blood Glucose: _____

Target Morning Fasting Blood Glucose: _____

Use your doctor's binder to find this information from your last checkup:

Current HbA1c: _____

If your A1c is above 7.0%, record your current bedtime blood glucose: _____

Current Blood Pressure: _____

Current Blood Triglyceride: _____

Current HDL Cholesterol and LDL Cholesterol: _____

---

**KEEP A WATCH FOR METABOLIC SYNDROME**

As you optimize your circadian rhythm by adopting IF, a reasonable goal is to reverse all your numbers so that you can avoid both diabetes and its metabolic syndrome sinister friends. All these numbers can be reversed:

- High levels of blood glucose
- Abdominal obesity
- High blood pressure
- High triglycerides
- High-density lipoprotein cholesterol (HDLC) levels

---

## HOW DO YOU FEEL?

The goal of optimizing your circadian rhythm is to improve both your daily sense of wellness and your laboratory test numbers. When you can quantify feeling better along your journey to improved laboratory numbers, then you are more likely to continue the journey well past the 12-week challenge.

Use the following grid to record your scores on a scale of 1 to 10. Refer to the assessments in Chapter 4 to see which symptoms are bothering you most. Use my prompts to accurately target your response. Or, imagine how you felt when you were completely healthy and fit; that may have been in your teenage years or your 20s or 30s. Think of that as your best score (a score of 10) and then imagine how you feel now compared to your personal best. Here's the key for using the grid.

1. **Morning pain and stiffness:** 1 = significant pain whereby you cannot function normally for up to an hour after waking up; 10 = no pain in any joint and no stiffness.
2. **Morning energy:** 1 = chronic morning fatigue; 10 = full of energy.
3. **Daytime mental clarity:** 1 = inability to stay on task and/or remember tasks; 10 = competent and clear-headed.
4. **Energy after physical activity:** 1 = cannot walk up two flights of stairs without losing breath or feeling very tired after a few minutes of working in the backyard or moderate physical activity; 10 = little or no sense of physical tiredness even after an hour of brisk walking or jogging.
5. **Aches and pains (headaches, back pain, joint pain, etc.):** 1 = experiencing any of these pains at least once a day and you take medication to find relief; 10 = an entire week free from aches and pains.
6. **Mood:** 1= feeling low, pessimistic about the future, anxious; 10 = happy, upbeat, and hopeful.
7. **Hunger:** 1 = excessive hunger pangs at least twice a day outside of meals; 10 = no feeling of extreme hunger outside of meals throughout the day or night.
8. **Gut health:** 1 = bloated, gas, heartburn, indigestion, irregular bowel movement; 10 = none of these symptoms on any day of the past week.
9. **Bedtime sleepiness:** 1 = not tired at bedtime, taking more than 30 minutes in bed to fall asleep; 10 = tired and ready to fall asleep in 15 minutes.
10. **Sleep:** 1 = waking up two or three (or more) times and/or inability to stay asleep; 10 = at least 6 hours of uninterrupted sleep or waking up only once to use the bathroom or to sip some water.

| How I Feel Before the Program | Scale of 1 to 10 |
|---|---|
| **1.** Morning pain and stiffness | |
| **2.** Morning energy | |
| **3.** Daytime mental clarity | |
| **4.** Energy after physical activity | |
| **5.** Aches and pains | |
| **6.** Mood | |
| **7.** Hunger | |
| **8.** Gut health | |
| **9.** Bedtime sleepiness | |
| **10.** Sleep | |

## START THE 12-WEEK CHALLENGE

We typically start our challenge participants on a Friday or the last day of their workweek. We find that this is the best day to go to bed early after your first day of IF. And if you cannot get to sleep because of hunger or a headache, you have the opportunity to sleep in on Saturday morning. If you can avoid a Friday-night feast on your first attempt, you will overcome one of the major hurdles in adopting IF.

Record your results on page 232 and in your notebook:

## WEEKS 1 AND 2: FOCUS ON A 12-HOUR IF

1. Food timing. Choose your 12-hour window for eating all your meals. Follow all the guidelines in Chapter 5 to determine the 12 hours that will best fit your existing lifestyle and how many meals you will eat.

2. Sleep time. Set a time that you can be in bed each night. The goal is to spend at least 7 hours in bed every night.

3. Set your night-light/night shift features on all computer screens and your smartphone to make the screens dim and turn orange 2 hours before your bedtime. This will be your nudge to get ready for sleep.

4. Adjust your bedroom temperature to 70°F or lower at night. Use the bathroom before going to bed, so that you don't wake up to use the bathroom at night. After waking up in the morning, make it a point to open the window curtains to let the daylight flood into your room.

5. Go outside after waking up to get some daylight for roughly 15 minutes. You can go for a short walk or do stretching exercise outdoors.

6. Plan your food for the day, including when you will eat and what you will eat, and prepare accordingly. Pack a lunch and snack, if necessary.

7. Remove the "no" foods listed in Chapter 6 from your home. Otherwise, follow your typical diet.

8. If you don't currently exercise at all, start the exercise program with stretches. Use the internet to locate online stretching exercises or yoga classes you can follow. I like the program outlined in the book *Vital Yoga*, by Meta Hirschl. If you currently exercise, follow the schedule outlined in Chapter 7, moving your exercise time to afternoon and/or early evening, which is better for managing blood glucose than exercise in the morning. If you cannot find time in the afternoon or evening, exercise whenever you have time.

9. Record your weekly weight and daily morning fasting blood glucose reading.

10. Record the results for the "How I Feel" survey at the end of the week.

## WEEKS 3 AND 4: SWITCH TO A 10-HOUR IF

1.  Food timing. Condense your eating window to 10 hours that best fit your lifestyle. Follow all the guidelines in Chapter 5 to determine the 10 hours that will best fit your existing lifestyle and how many meals you will eat.

2.  Sleep. Avoid sleeping with pets or people who wake up at night. Train your children to sleep in their own beds. If you have a snoring partner, start using a pair of comfortable earplugs. If you cannot make the bedroom completely dark, try an eye mask.

3.  Push your first cup of coffee or tea to your new breakfast time. If you must have a hot beverage as soon as you wake up, try hot water with lemon juice or a decaffeinated herbal tea. Enjoy your coffee with milk and one of the approved sweeteners with breakfast.

4.  Increase your breakfast size to make it the biggest meal of the day.

5.  Have no coffee, tea, or hot chocolate after 2:00 p.m. to ensure that you will get a good night's sleep. If you are feeling low in energy in the afternoon, have a large glass of water.

6.  Swap out packaged energy bars for nuts, hummus, fresh raw vegetables, and fruit as a snack.

7.  Check your step count before dinner. Make a target of reaching 5,000 steps every day. If your step count is low, plan to go for a walk after dinner.

8.  Add strength training to your stretching routine. Use the internet to find an online strength training exercise program that you can do in the comfort of your home. Follow the schedule set up in Chapter 7. You will be doing strength exercises only two days a week, with three days off in between to let your body adjust.

9.  Record your weekly weight and daily morning fasting blood glucose reading.

10. Record the results for the "How I Feel" survey at the end of the week.

## WEEKS 5 AND 6: FOCUS ON FOOD QUALITY

1.  Food timing. Pay closer attention to how hungry you feel during your 10-hour IF. If you don't feel hungry between breakfast and lunch, then your body has fully adjusted to the new eating window. You do not have to snack between meals. Think of snacks as an emergency option.

2.  Use the shopping list in Chapter 6 when you go to the grocer. Try five or ten new food items from the list to use in preparing new Mediterranean diet recipes.

3.  Focus on lunch and dinner. Decrease the sizes of lunch and dinner per the instructions in Chapter 5. Pay attention to specific food recommendations for each of these meals to create a daily balanced diet.

4.  Continue with your stretching and weight training exercises. Add in aerobic exercise, following the schedule in Chapter 7. For the best benefit and least risk for injury, try doing all your exercise in the afternoon, either before or after dinner.

5.  Add 5 to 10 minutes of physical activity after dinner. It does not have to be immediately after eating; you can wait for 15 to 30 minutes and then go for a walk around the block, or climb three or four flights of stairs (holding the rail, so that you don't fall), or get on an elliptical or treadmill. If you can do your aerobic exercise only once a day, do it after dinner, but not within 1 hour of bedtime. If you can only exercise close to bedtime, take a tepid shower to cool down so that you can sleep well.

6.  Sleep time. Increase your time in bed to 8 hours every night.

7.  If you are still struggling with falling asleep, try some of the strategies discussed in Chapter 8 (evening bath, relaxation techniques, etc.).

8.  Stay hydrated to aid in digestion, improve your energy levels throughout the day, and avoid headaches. There's no such thing as drinking too much water.

9.  Record your weekly weight and daily morning fasting blood glucose reading.
10. Record the results for the "How I Feel" survey at the end of the week.

## WEEKS 7 AND 8: DON'T LET YOUR GUARD DOWN

1.  After six weeks, many people hit a hurdle, feeling tired of being rigorous with IF or wanting to "reward" themselves for their success by cheating a little. Don't let that happen. It will only set back your ultimate success.
2.  It's okay to eat less if you find that you are not hungry at your set mealtimes. In fact, one of the most effective ways to manage diabetes is to reduce your total calorie intake.
3.  Review the foods you have been eating and see if you can make adjustments by eating more fresh fruits and vegetables and lean protein, and less low-GI packaged foods like bread, rice, and pasta.
4.  Try a new cuisine that adheres to the tenets of the Mediterranean diet. There are hundreds of cookbooks that focus on Italian, Middle Eastern, Greek, and Moroccan foods. Or, see if you can adapt any of your old favorites with healthier, low-GI ingredients.
5.  Exercise does not have to be just brisk walking and structured exercise. Household chores, working in the garden, or volunteering for a good cause all involve physical activity. Try to substitute your structured aerobic exercise time with one of these for at least one day a week. It can reduce your stress and provide a sense of achievement.
6.  Keep working on achieving better sleep. Try relaxing meditation music to help you unwind and fall asleep.
7.  Record your weekly weight and daily morning fasting blood glucose reading.
8.  Record the results for the "How I Feel" survey at the end of the week.

## WEEKS 9 AND 10: TAKING IF ON THE ROAD

1. Prepare to start eating outside of the home. Plan for communal meals that work with your food lists and eating schedule.

2. Choose restaurants that feature Italian, Middle Eastern, Greek, or Moroccan foods. If the portions are larger than you have become accustomed to, take home half or share them family style.

3. Discuss your progress and challenges with your family or friends. Your positive experience may even inspire your family and friends to adopt IF and keep you company on your IF journey.

4. If you are feeling comfortable with your resistance exercise, it may be time to take it up a notch. Add more repetitions and/or increase the resistance. Focus on new muscle groups.

5. Improve your travel sleep by bringing a comfortable neck pillow, eye mask, earplugs, and a nose strip/nose clip for on the road. In flight, you can more easily doze off with this gear, and in a new hotel room or bedroom, the eye mask and earplugs can be handy if there is too much light or too much noise.

6. Schedule your next doctor's visit and lab work for after completion of the 12-week challenge. Ask to have your fasting glucose, HbA1c, cholesterol, and blood pressure checked.

7. Record your weekly weight and daily morning fasting blood glucose reading.

8. Record the results for the "How I Feel" survey at the end of the week.

## WEEKS 11 AND 12: THE HOME STRETCH

1. Eating good-quality food should not break the bank. Consider becoming a member of a food coop or shop at stores that sell in bulk—such as Costco—to buy whole-grain flour, olive oil, dried beans, tofu, fish, meats, eggs, milk, yogurt, cheese, peanuts, almonds, spar-

kling water, vegetables, and fruits. Your area may have a local farmers' market. Another good resource is ethnic stores, like Asian markets, which often have many fresh vegetables, tofu, fish at a better price, or new options to try.

2.  Move all your exercise to the afternoon or evening, with an additional walk after dinner.

3.  It is okay to nap for an hour during the day. Don't nap too much, as that will make it difficult to fall asleep at your habitual bedtime.

4.  If you are still struggling with getting the right amount of sleep, try eliminating coffee, tea, and dark chocolate for a week. Observe if you are sleeping more or falling into a deeper sleep. This is a sign that you may have to reduce your caffeine intake to get the sleep that your body needs.

5.  Record your weekly weight and daily morning fasting blood glucose reading.

6.  Record the results for the "How I Feel" survey at the end of the week.

## CHART YOUR PROGRESS

If you cannot monitor something, you cannot manage it. Every day, you will write down the details of your new circadian rhythm. It may sound burdensome, but you will spend less than five minutes a day recording your experience, and you'll be able to instantly see your progress. Each time you answer yes to a question on the chart, give yourself 1 point. A perfect score each day is 6 points. Over time, see how you are making improvements to your score by aligning your eating, sleeping, and exercising to your circadian code.

## PROGRESS CHARTS FOR 12-WEEK CHALLENGE

| Weeks 1-2 | Did you sleep for at least 7 hours? | After waking up, did you wait for at least 1 hour before eating or drinking something with calories? | Did you eat all your food and beverages (except water) within 12 hours? | Did you get outdoors for at least 30 minutes during the day? | Did you exercise or walk briskly for at least 30 minutes? | Did you stop eating and dim the lights ≥ 2 hours before bedtime? | TOTAL DAILY SCORE (OUT OF 6) |
|---|---|---|---|---|---|---|---|
| Mon | | | | | | | |
| Tues | | | | | | | |
| Wed | | | | | | | |
| Thurs | | | | | | | |
| Fri | | | | | | | |
| Sat | | | | | | | |
| Sun | | | | | | | |
| Total week 1 score | | | | | | | |
| Mon | | | | | | | |
| Tues | | | | | | | |
| Wed | | | | | | | |
| Thurs | | | | | | | |
| Fri | | | | | | | |
| Sat | | | | | | | |
| Sun | | | | | | | |
| Total week 2 score | | | | | | | |

| Weeks 3-4 | Did you sleep for at least 7 hours? | After waking up, did you wait for at least 1 hour before eating or drinking something with calories? | Did you eat all your food and beverages (except water) within 12 hours? | Did you get outdoors for at least 30 minutes during the day? | Did you exercise or walk briskly for at least 30 minutes? | Did you stop eating and dim the lights ≥ 2 hours before bedtime? | Total daily score (out of 6) |
|---|---|---|---|---|---|---|---|
| Mon | | | | | | | |
| Tues | | | | | | | |
| Wed | | | | | | | |
| Thurs | | | | | | | |
| Fri | | | | | | | |
| Sat | | | | | | | |
| Sun | | | | | | | |
| Total week 3 score | | | | | | | |
| Mon | | | | | | | |
| Tues | | | | | | | |
| Wed | | | | | | | |
| Thurs | | | | | | | |
| Fri | | | | | | | |
| Sat | | | | | | | |
| Sun | | | | | | | |
| Total week 4 score | | | | | | | |

| Weeks 5-6 | Did you sleep for at least 7 hours? | After waking up, did you wait for at least 1 hour before eating or drinking something with calories? | Did you eat all your food and beverages (except water) within 12 hours? | Did you get outdoors for at least 30 minutes during the day? | Did you exercise or walk briskly for at least 30 minutes? | Did you stop eating and dim the lights ≥ 2 hours before bedtime? | Total daily score (out of 6) |
|---|---|---|---|---|---|---|---|
| Mon | | | | | | | |
| Tues | | | | | | | |
| Wed | | | | | | | |
| Thurs | | | | | | | |
| Fri | | | | | | | |
| Sat | | | | | | | |
| Sun | | | | | | | |
| Total week 5 score | | | | | | | |
| Mon | | | | | | | |
| Tues | | | | | | | |
| Wed | | | | | | | |
| Thurs | | | | | | | |
| Fri | | | | | | | |
| Sat | | | | | | | |
| Sun | | | | | | | |
| Total week 6 score | | | | | | | |

| Weeks 7-8 | Did you sleep for at least 7 hours? | After waking up, did you wait for at least 1 hour before eating or drinking something with calories? | Did you eat all your food and beverages (except water) within 12 hours? | Did you get outdoors for at least 30 minutes during the day? | Did you exercise or walk briskly for at least 30 minutes? | Did you stop eating and dim the lights ≥ 2 hours before bedtime? | Total daily score (out of 6) |
|---|---|---|---|---|---|---|---|
| Mon | | | | | | | |
| Tues | | | | | | | |
| Wed | | | | | | | |
| Thurs | | | | | | | |
| Fri | | | | | | | |
| Sat | | | | | | | |
| Sun | | | | | | | |
| Total week 7 . score | | | | | | | |
| Mon | | | | | | | |
| Tues | | | | | | | |
| Wed | | | | | | | |
| Thurs | | | | | | | |
| Fri | | | | | | | |
| Sat | | | | | | | |
| Sun | | | | | | | |
| Total week 8 score | | | | | | | |

| Weeks 9-10 | Did you sleep for at least 7 hours? | After waking up, did you wait for at least 1 hour before eating or drinking something with calories? | Did you eat all your food and beverages (except water) within 12 hours? | Did you get outdoors for at least 30 minutes during the day? | Did you exercise or walk briskly for at least 30 minutes? | Did you stop eating and dim the lights ≥ 2 hours before bedtime? | Total daily score (out of 6) |
|---|---|---|---|---|---|---|---|
| Mon | | | | | | | |
| Tues | | | | | | | |
| Wed | | | | | | | |
| Thurs | | | | | | | |
| Fri | | | | | | | |
| Sat | | | | | | | |
| Sun | | | | | | | |
| Total week 9 score | | | | | | | |
| Mon | | | | | | | |
| Tues | | | | | | | |
| Wed | | | | | | | |
| Thurs | | | | | | | |
| Fri | | | | | | | |
| Sat | | | | | | | |
| Sun | | | | | | | |
| Total week 10 score | | | | | | | |

| Weeks 11–12 | Did you sleep for at least 7 hours? | After waking up, did you wait for at least 1 hour before eating or drinking something with calories? | Did you eat all your food and beverages (except water) within 12 hours? | Did you get outdoors for at least 30 minutes during the day? | Did you exercise or walk briskly for at least 30 minutes? | Did you stop eating and dim the lights ≥ 2 hours before bedtime? | Total daily score (out of 6) |
|---|---|---|---|---|---|---|---|
| Mon | | | | | | | |
| Tues | | | | | | | |
| Wed | | | | | | | |
| Thurs | | | | | | | |
| Fri | | | | | | | |
| Sat | | | | | | | |
| Sun | | | | | | | |
| Total week 11 score | | | | | | | |
| Mon | | | | | | | |
| Tues | | | | | | | |
| Wed | | | | | | | |
| Thurs | | | | | | | |
| Fri | | | | | | | |
| Sat | | | | | | | |
| Sun | | | | | | | |
| Total week 12 score | | | | | | | |

## HAS MY HEALTH CHANGED?

In addition to using the progress charts, you can track how the rest of your health is changing. Over the next 12 weeks, use the following chart to record how you feel in each of the same categories at the end of the week. The goal is to see these numbers shift upward so that by Week 12, all your numbers are closer to 10. It may take a week or so before you notice if your health, mood, or energy improves. You might also see that you hit a plateau, then overcome it later. This is a very typical pattern we've found in our studies.

| How I Feel During the 12-Week Challenge | | | | | | | | | | | | |
|---|---|---|---|---|---|---|---|---|---|---|---|---|
| Weeks ▸ | 1 | 2 | 3 | 4 | 5 | 6 | 7 | 8 | 9 | 10 | 11 | 12 |
| 1. Morning pain and stiffness | | | | | | | | | | | | |
| 2. Morning energy | | | | | | | | | | | | |
| 3. Daytime mental clarity | | | | | | | | | | | | |
| 4. Energy after physical activity | | | | | | | | | | | | |
| 5. Aches and pains | | | | | | | | | | | | |
| 6. Mood | | | | | | | | | | | | |
| 7. Hunger | | | | | | | | | | | | |
| 8. Gut health | | | | | | | | | | | | |
| 9. Bedtime sleepiness | | | | | | | | | | | | |
| 10. Sleep | | | | | | | | | | | | |

## MEET KOFI

Throughout this book, you've met many of my study participants and friends, and even my mother. This time, I introduce you to my friend Kofi, a shift worker who lives in my neighborhood. His story reflects every aspect of aligning one's life with one's circadian rhythm. The changes Kofi has gone through are subtle but powerful. And you can see how the whole program works by following his journey.

Kofi was 36 years old when he was diagnosed with diabetes. He remembers the day vividly, because he never expected to hear his doctor say, "Kofi, you're not doing too well taking care of yourself." His HbA1c was 6.6%, and his fasting blood glucose was 132 mg/dL.

Kofi always knew he was at high risk for developing diabetes. As an African American man who had a family history of heart disease and diabetes, he had too many risk factors to allow himself the freedom of not worrying about his health. He worked with his doctor to create an aggressive plan to control his blood glucose, and he started taking metformin right away. He was hoping that the medication would help him slow the disease, yet in just a few years it became progressively worse. By the time he was 48, the metformin alone was not enough to control his diabetes: in just 12 years, his HbA1c had shot up to 8%, which was a sign that he was heading straight toward heart disease. This time, the doctor recommended adding another medication (metformin twice daily and glipizide once a day). Yet after living with diabetes for 15 years, by his fifty-first birthday, even with two meds, his HbA1c was 7.6%. So, his doctor added a statin drug to control his blood cholesterol, had him take vitamin $B_{12}$ to counter the effects of the metformin, and recommended a few over-the-counter aids for his occasional stomach upset. The cholesterol-lowering drug could also make him feel muscle pain once in a while, so he picked up an extra bottle of Advil.

As long as I've known Kofi, he has tried to eat healthy; he had long ago swapped soda for fruit juice; avoided white bread; ate healthy snack bars, bran breakfast cereals, and low-fat milk; and limited his eating of rice to once a day. He would occasionally walk in our neighborhood in the evening or during weekends. He often complained to me that he would get extremely hungry in the afternoon, to the point where he had a snack that was almost as big as a meal. At least once a week, he would wake up at night with hypoglycemia and had to chug a large glass of orange juice. Kofi also complained about sleep problems, which are pretty common among shift workers. It seemed like it was always difficult for him to get a good night's sleep.

He was convinced that he had done the best he could to change his lifestyle, and that this gradual slide in his health was what should be expected with diabetes. A few of his friends were also living with diabetes for 15 years, were less careful about their diets and exercise, and were in worse shape. Two of them were taking daily insulin shots, and one had already suffered kidney damage.

One day I was telling him about a new study I was working on that specifically looked at firefighters and IF. Kofi was intrigued, and he thought he had nothing to lose by signing up. After a consultation with his endocrinologist, he stopped taking the glipizide, as this could reduce his blood sugar to dangerously low levels while he was doing a 10-hour IF. Part of the study was to keep careful notes, so we have a complete record of his experience. Here it is:

WEEK 1. Prior to IF, Kofi would wake up at 4:00 a.m. and immediately have a cup of coffee with milk and sugar to completely wake up. An hour or so later, he would eat breakfast. He would pack lunch some days to take to work. He usually came back home at 3:00 p.m. when his shift was over, ate a meal, and then before going to bed would have a piece of fruit as a snack at 8:00 p.m. During the day he would also snack a few times—chewing on something "healthy" like a granola or protein bar.

On Day 1, Kofi recorded his morning fasting blood glucose 30 minutes after waking up, and it was 172 mg/dL. Way too high, and he jumped right into a 10-hour IF eating window of 8:00 a.m. to 6:00 p.m. The first week was hard, as he had hunger pangs after his last meal. His poor sleep felt worse than usual because he now had to deal with a hunger headache. After three days, his body revolted and he had to revert to a small snack after dinner, and that seemed to do the trick. His IF eating window was now roughly 11 hours.

WEEK 2. Kofi decided to go for a walk on Saturday morning by Lake Miramar. The walk around the lake is five miles, and he had never done such a long walk before. The walk took 1 hour 25 minutes, and when he was done, Kofi was tired. He realized that many of his joints were weak or painful. But he was happy that he could make it around the lake. By the end of Week 2, his nightly hunger pangs had subsided, and for the first time he was able to sleep for 6 hours, only waking up for a short time to go to the bathroom.

WEEKS 3 AND 4. Kofi decided to go back to a 10-hour IF. His Saturday morning walk around the lake was becoming less painful, yet it still took about the same amount of time. He also noticed that his morning blood glucose had come down slightly to between 160 and 170 mg/dL for 13 out of 14 days. One day, it was over 170 mg/dL. By the end of four weeks, his joint pain was almost gone. On Saturday and Sunday nights, he could sleep uninterrupted for 7 hours and he felt great the following mornings. He thought the reason may be a combination of IF, the long walks, and reduced stress.

WEEKS 5 TO 8. By Week 5, his new lifestyle felt normal, without any effort. There were no more hunger pangs, his joint pain had substantially reduced, his sleep was improving to the point where only two or three nights in a week Kofi would wake up at night. His mood was also getting better. His family noticed that he was more energetic even after a long shift of work. Best of all, his morning fasting glucose was now hovering between 140 and 150 mg/dL. Those were numbers he hadn't seen in years.

WEEKS 9 TO 12. My firefighter study ended after Week 12, but Kofi was able to stay on his new IF lifestyle while continuing to work the early-morning shift. He shaved off 10 minutes from his five miles around the lake. In fact, he was becoming quite competitive in walking and would feel bad if someone overtook him. He had also lost some weight. By this point, his fasting glucose was hovering between 130 and 140 mg/dL.

At the end of 12 weeks, when he got his lab tests done, he was surprised to see his HbA1c drop from 7.6 to 7.1%. He hadn't seen numbers so low in four years. In a simple sense, he had reversed his diabetes by four years, and he was able to achieve it even after getting off one diabetes medication. He was becoming a strong believer of "IF is medicine."

By this point, Kofi no longer had to keep records because the study was over. But he liked the sense of control that knowing his numbers provided. In fact, he had started taking his blood glucose reading 30 minutes after lunch or dinner, as well as before breakfast. Sometimes he was surprised to see readings as high as 220 mg/dL. He thought there was still room for improvement when it came to making good food choices, and that he could lower his blood sugar even more. So, he convinced his endocrinologist to prescribe him a CGM.

Although Kofi's wife, June, had perfect blood sugar levels, she was slightly overweight and was mildly hypertensive, with a blood pressure reading of 130/85. She never wanted to take a blood pressure medication. She also wanted to try IF to lose some weight and improve her blood pressure. So, she joined Kofi in his IF. She didn't have to check her blood sugar and didn't want to check her blood pressure every day. She just wanted to step on the scale every week. Kofi was thrilled that they would do IF together.

WEEKS 13 TO 16. After putting the CGM on, Kofi was like a kid at a science fair. After every meal he would check his blood glucose to see how it rose, how long it stayed up, and how long it took to resume a normal level. The first week was an eye-opener for him. Almost every "healthy" cereal and wheat bread he had in his cabinet was causing sugar spikes above 200 mg/dL. The healthy snack bars were no exception. A post-snack glucose as high as 180 mg/dL was common. He also realized that none of his fruit juice choices were actually healthy. Everything he ate or drank was spiking his glucose above 160 mg/dL.

He started to experiment with almost everything he was eating. He would look up the glycemic index of foods on the web and check his CGM after eating them. It became a glucose game for him. After testing homemade meals, packaged foods, snacks, and beverages, he came to a simple conclusion: the food items that came in ready-to-eat packages were not good for him. The bread, pasta, and rice he ate daily were also not that good for his blood sugar levels. It was one thing to be told which foods may not be good for diabetes, and it was another to experience first-hand how his blood sugar was reacting. The CGM became his best friend.

He also started experimenting with his exercise routine. One day, 30 minutes after finishing his dinner, he went for a walk around the block. His post-dinner glucose reading had gone up to 200 mg/dL. But after just 15 minutes on his walk, his blood glucose reading started to go down, and in the next 30 minutes it reached 140. This was significantly different from his typical post-dinner reading, when his glucose would remain around 200 and would take almost two or three hours before going down to 140. He repeated the walking experiment the next day, and he got a similar result. He tried it after lunch; same result. Just 15 minutes of brisk walking after a big meal was as effective as taking a diabetes pill. The walk became his new routine. Instead of looking forward to a post-dinner snack, he was eager for his post-dinner walk and checking on his CGM.

By the end of 16 weeks (and just 4 weeks of wearing the CGM), Kofi noticed that on the days in which he ate healthy and did some brisk walking, his blood sugar throughout the day would rarely go above 180 mg/dL and his morning blood glucose would be below 130. On one day, he could not believe his glucose reading in the morning—119 mg/dL. He checked again with a finger-prick glucose reading and it was very close—121. He was ecstatic. In his 15 years of living with diabetes, he had never seen a lab glucose test or at-home morning fasting blood glucose reading of 120 mg/dL.

Waking up in the middle of the night and failing to go back to sleep was a thing of the past. He also started some resistance training at home using free weights and his body as weight (push-ups, sit-ups, planks, etc.). He tried to do at least 10 minutes of stretching before or after his resistance training and his weekend walk around the lake.

WEEKS 17 TO 20. Kofi was now focused on changing what he ate and preparing most of his meals at home. Instead of buying bread from the store, he bought stone-ground whole wheat flour and started baking his own low-glycemic bread. Similarly, he switched to whole wheat pasta and parboiled or brown rice as his main starches. For breakfast, he would enjoy his homemade bread with a slice of avocado, a slice of cheese, and a hard-boiled egg or an omelet. For lunch, he switched between a salad and a small grilled fillet of fish, grilled mushrooms, or tofu and a side of sautéed or grilled vegetables, or a bowl of lentil soup with a cup of brown rice topped with butter. His family dinners became quite small and consisted typically of some meat sautéed in olive oil with fresh vegetables. His old store-bought snacks were mostly gone. His new snacks were in-shell roasted and unsalted peanuts, edamame, dried figs, homemade hummus and baby carrots/celery sticks/cucumber, and roasted almonds. He and his wife June started to make their own yogurt and cottage cheese at home, and they found that it would last almost the entire week and tasted much better than the store-bought versions. And surprisingly, Kofi found eating healthy by preparing meals at home was actually cheaper than eating out or eating packaged foods.

WEEKS 21 TO 24. By the end of Week 20, Kofi had a new life. His general sense about diabetes had flipped from diabetes being in charge of his life to his being in charge of his blood sugar. He started dreaming about what he would do beyond 60 or 65 years of age. He called his doctor to schedule new labs for the end of 24 weeks.

By Week 23, he could finish the five-mile loop in 55 minutes, and afterward he didn't feel tired at all and was ready for the second lap. His daily step count was up to 7,000 steps a day. He realized that he had more muscle pain and sore joints when he was sedentary. Even though he was walking more these days, he barely had any muscle pain. He felt he was 10 to 15 years younger.

After 24 weeks, when he got his lab results, they proved that his biological clock had literally dialed back his diabetes by 12 years. His fasting blood glucose came out at 126 mg/dL, and HbA1c was 6.8%—

the number he had ten years ago. But more than that, he was sleeping better, feeling more energetic, had less body pain, and was happier than before. He was at his best weight—134 pounds. His cholesterol had also come down to a point where his doctor recommended that he reduce his cholesterol medication by half.

As his family continued with their IF, his wife also lost a few pounds and her blood pressure became normal. They chose to celebrate their new healthy life with new clothes—both Kofi and June had lost enough belly fat that they dropped a whole pants size.

Although he cannot go back in time and erase diabetes from his health history, Kofi is insisting that his son, who is 18 years old, and his daughter, who is 16 years old, start getting their fasting blood glucose and HbA1c tests done every year at their annual health checkups. He is also hoping that the new circadian lifestyle that his family has adopted will give his children years of a healthy and productive life.

## FINAL THOUGHTS

Kofi's story isn't unique. In fact, it's more the rule than the exception for our study participants. Now you can see the same results by working in alignment with this new lifestyle.

Circadian science is new, and the breakthroughs we are finding are helping people live many additional years, with much better health. It is becoming apparent that when people follow IF diligently, and they combine it with an optimum circadian rhythm, they can see multiple benefits beyond glucose control. Every day, we are learning that an optimum circadian rhythm, practiced through IF and the many other suggestions I've made in this book, has numerous benefits for various organ systems, the body's immune system, and the brain. Scientists from all over the world and all leading funding agencies are recognizing the untapped potential of a healthy circadian rhythm, either alone or in combination with medication, as the best approach to prevent, manage, and reverse a wide range of diseases, from cancer to dementia. We will know soon whether IF, with an optimum circadian code, is the multi-solving magic bullet for good health.

## THE COMPLETE BENEFITS OF OPTIMIZING YOUR CIRCADIAN CODE

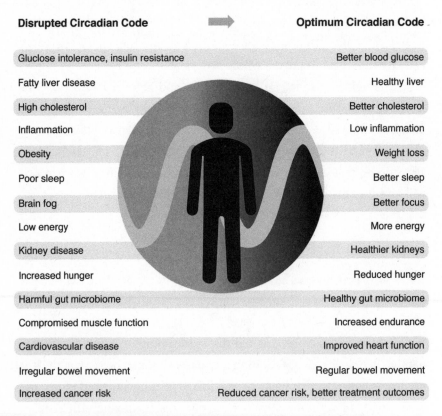

| Disrupted Circadian Code | Optimum Circadian Code |
|---|---|
| Gluclose intolerance, insulin resistance | Better blood glucose |
| Fatty liver disease | Healthy liver |
| High cholesterol | Better cholesterol |
| Inflammation | Low inflammation |
| Obesity | Weight loss |
| Poor sleep | Better sleep |
| Brain fog | Better focus |
| Low energy | More energy |
| Kidney disease | Healthier kidneys |
| Increased hunger | Reduced hunger |
| Harmful gut microbiome | Healthy gut microbiome |
| Compromised muscle function | Increased endurance |
| Cardiovascular disease | Improved heart function |
| Irregular bowel movement | Regular bowel movement |
| Increased cancer risk | Reduced cancer risk, better treatment outcomes |

Complete benefits of living with optimum circadian code by adopting a 10-hour intermittent fasting, sleep discipline, and daily exercise.

In the meantime, we do know that diabetes is a silent pandemic raging throughout the world, and it is the cause of a specific downward spiral of health that ultimately ends in heart disease, stroke, liver disease, cancer, kidney failure, or dementia. Diabetes also makes it easy for infectious diseases like COVID-19 to do terrible damage to the body and brain. Yet when IF and better circadian alignment is practiced over a few months, people can retrain the liver and fat tissues to break down unwanted fat and cholesterol, reversing liver disease. In preclinical studies, we have found a clear sign of a reduction in risk for heart disease. We are also finding that IF improves kidney function.

I thank you for following along with my research, and I hope you will start implementing this program today. Then you will join the thousands of people all over the world who are taking their health into their own hands. All you need to do is follow your natural code. It's time for you to experience the IF difference for yourself. I sincerely wish you luck as you begin this journey to reach the best health of your life.

# NOTES

## CHAPTER 1

1.  Emerging Risk Factors Collaboration, Sarwar N, Gao P, Seshasai SR, Gobin R, Kaptoge S, Di Angelantonio E, Ingelsson E, Lawlor DA, Selvin E, Stampfer M, Stehouwer CD, Lewington S, Pennells L, Thompson A, Sattar N, White IR, Ray KK, Danesh J. Diabetes mellitus, fasting blood glucose concentration, and risk of vascular disease: a collaborative meta-analysis of 102 prospective studies. *Lancet.* 2010 Jun 26;375(9733):2215–22. doi: 10.1016/S0140-6736(10)60484-9. Erratum in: *Lancet.* 2010 Sep 18;376(9745):958. Hillage HL [corrected to Hillege HL].
2.  https://www.cdc.gov/diabetes/basics/index.html.
3.  https://www.heart.org/en/health-topics/diabetes/why-diabetes-matters/cardio vascular-disease—diabetes.
4.  https://spectrum.diabetesjournals.org/content/27/4/276.
5.  Li S, Williams PL, Douglass CW. Development of a clinical guideline to predict undiagnosed diabetes in dental patients. *J Am Dent Assoc.* 2011 Jan;142(1):28–37. doi: 10.14219/jada.archive.2011.0025.
6.  Diabetes and depression: Coping with the two conditions—Mayo Clinic, www .mayoclinic.org/diseases-conditions/diabetes/expert-answers/diabetes-and -depression/faq-20057904.
7.  https://dermnetnz.org/topics/diabetic-foot-ulcer.
8.  Thong EP, Codner E, Laven JSE, Teede H. Diabetes: a metabolic and reproductive disorder in women. *Lancet Diabetes Endocrinol.* 2020 Feb;8(2):134–49. doi: 10.1016/ S2213-8587(19)30345-6. Epub 2019 Oct 18.

## CHAPTER 2

1.  Konopka RJ, Benzer S. Clock mutants of Drosophila melanogaster. *Proc Nat Acad Sci USA.* 1971;68(9):2112–16. doi:10.1073/pnas.68.9.2112.
2.  Mure LS, Le HD, Benegiamo G, Chang MW, Rios L, Jillani N, Ngotho M, Kariuki T, Dkhissi-Benyahya O, Cooper HM, Panda S. Diurnal transcriptome atlas of a primate across major neural and peripheral tissues. *Science.* 2018 Mar 16;359(6381):eaao0318. doi: 10.1126/science.aao0318. Epub 2018 Feb 8.
3.  Panda S et al. Coordinated transcription of key pathways in the mouse by the circadian clock. *Cell* 2002;109(3):307–20.
4.  Coomans CP, van den Berg SA, Lucassen EA, Houben T, Pronk AC, van der Spek RD, Kalsbeek A, Biermasz NR, Willems van Dijk K, Romijn JA, Meijer JH. The

suprachiasmatic nucleus controls circadian energy metabolism and hepatic insulin sensitivity. *Diabetes.* 2013 Apr;62(4):1102–08. doi: 10.2337/db12-0507. Epub 2012 Dec 28.

5. Chaix A, Panda S. Ketone bodies signal opportunistic food-seeking activity. *Trends Endocrinol Metab.* 2016 Jun;27(6):350–52. doi: 10.1016/j.tem.2016.03.014. Epub 2016 Mar 30.

6. Puchalska P, Crawford PA. Multi-dimensional roles of ketone bodies in fuel metabolism, signaling, and therapeutics. *Cell Metab.* 2017 Feb 7;25(2):262–84. doi: 10.1016/j.cmet.2016.12.022.

7. Wilmsen EN. Studies in diet, nutrition, and fertility among a group of Kalahari Bushmen in Botswana. *Social Science Information.* 1982;21(1):95–125. doi:10.1177/053901882021001006.

8. Boulos Z, Terman M. Food availability and daily biological rhythms. *Neurosci Biobehav Rev* 1980;4(2):119–31. doi:10.1016/0149-7634(80)90010-x.

9. Vollmers C et al. Time of feeding and the intrinsic circadian clock drive rhythms in hepatic gene expression. *Proc Nat Acad Sci USA.* 2009;106(50):21453–58.

10. Gill S, Panda S. A smartphone app reveals erratic diurnal eating patterns in humans that can be modulated for health benefits. *Cell Metab.* 2015 Nov 3;22(5):789–98. doi: 10.1016/j.cmet.2015.09.005. Epub 2015 Sep 24.

11. Sandhu A, Milan S, Gurm HS. Daylight savings time and myocardial infarction. *Open Heart* 2014;1(1):e000019.

12. Eckel RH, Depner CM, Perreault L, Markwald RR, Smith MR, McHill AW, Higgins J, Melanson EL, Wright KP Jr. Morning circadian misalignment during short sleep duration impacts insulin sensitivity. *Curr Biol.* 2015 Nov 16;25(22):3004–10. doi: 10.1016/j.cub.2015.10.011. Epub 2015 Nov 5.

13. McHill AW, Wright KP Jr. Role of sleep and circadian disruption on energy expenditure and in metabolic predisposition to human obesity and metabolic disease. *Obes Rev.* 2017 Feb;18 Suppl 1:15–24. doi: 10.1111/obr.12503.

14. Knutsson A, Kempe A. Shift work and diabetes—a systematic review. *Chronobiol Int.* 2014 Dec;31(10):1146–51. doi: 10.3109/07420528.2014.957308. Epub 2014 Oct 7.

## CHAPTER 3

1. Chaix A, Lin T, Le HD, Chang MW, Panda S. Time-Restricted Feeding Prevents Obesity and Metabolic Syndrome in Mice Lacking a Circadian Clock. *Cell Metab.* 2019 Feb 5;29(2):303–319.e4. doi: 10.1016/j.cmet.2018.08.004. Epub 2018 Aug 30.

2. Morikawa Y, Nakagawa H, Miura K, Soyama Y, Ishizaki M, Kido T, Naruse Y, Suwazono Y, Nogawa K. Shift work and the risk of diabetes mellitus among Japanese male factory workers. *Scand J Work Environ Health.* 2005 Jun;31(3):179–83. doi: 10.5271/sjweh.867.

3. Toshihiro M, Saito K, Takikawa S, Takebe N, Onoda T, Satoh J. Psychosocial factors are independent risk factors for the development of type 2 diabetes in Japanese workers with impaired fasting glucose and/or impaired glucose tolerance. *Diabet Med.* 2008 Oct;25(10):1211–17. doi: 10.1111/j.1464-5491.2008.02566.x.

4. Scheer FA, Hilton MF, Mantzoros CS, Shea SA. Adverse metabolic and cardio-vascular consequences of circadian misalignment. *Proc Nat Acad Sci USA.* 2009 Mar 17;106(11):44538. doi: 10.1073/pnas.0808180106. Epub 2009 Mar 2.

5. Eriksson AK, van den Donk M, Hilding A, Östenson CG. Work stress, sense of coherence, and risk of type 2 diabetes in a prospective study of middle-aged Swedish men and women. *Diabetes Care.* 2013 Sep;36(9):2683–89. doi: 10.2337/dc12-1738. Epub 2013 May 1.

6. Pan A, Schernhammer E, Sun Q et al. (2011). Rotating night shift work and risk of type 2 diabetes: two prospective cohort studies in women. *PloS Med.* 2011;8:e1001141.

7. Chalernvanichakom T, Sithisarankul P, Hiransuthikul N. Shift work and type 2 diabetic patients' health. *J Med Assoc Thai.* 2008;91:1093–96.

8. Dupuis J et al. New genetic loci implicated in fasting glucose homeostasis and their impact on type 2 diabetes risk. *Nat Genet.* 2010 Feb;42(2):105–16. doi: 10.1038/ng.520. Epub 2010 Jan 17. Erratum in: *Nat Genet.* 2010 May;42(5):464.

9. Prokopenko I et al. Variants in MTNR1B influence fasting glucose levels. *Nat Genet.* 2009 Jan;41(1):77–81. doi: 10.1038/ng.290. Epub 2008 Dec 7.

10. Lyssenko V, Nagorny CL, Erdos MR, Wierup N, Jonsson A, Spégel P, Bugliani M, Saxena R, Fex M, Pulizzi N, Isomaa B, Tuomi T, Nilsson P, Kuusisto J, Tuomilehto J, Boehnke M, Altshuler D, Sundler F, Eriksson JG, Jackson AU, Laakso M, Marchetti P, Watanabe RM, Mulder H, Groop L. Common variant in MTNR1B associated with increased risk of type 2 diabetes and impaired early insulin secretion. *Nat Genet.* 2009 Jan;41(1):82–88. doi: 10.1038/ng.288. Epub 2008 Dec 7.

11. Bouatia-Naji N et al. A variant near MTNR1B is associated with increased fasting plasma glucose levels and type 2 diabetes risk. *Nat Genet.* 2009 Jan;41(1):89–94. doi: 10.1038/ng.277. Epub 2008 Dec 7.

12. Rönn T, Wen J, Yang Z, Lu B, Du Y, Groop L, Hu R, Ling C. A common variant in MTNR1B, encoding melatonin receptor 1B, is associated with type 2 diabetes and fasting plasma glucose in Han Chinese individuals. *Diabetologia.* 2009 May;52(5):830–33. doi: 10.1007/s00125-009-1297-8. Epub 2009 Feb 25.

13. Persaud SJ, Jones PM. A wake-up call for type 2 diabetes? *N Engl J Med.* 2016 Sep 15;375(11):1090–92. doi: 10.1056/NEJMcibr1607950.

14. Rudic RD, McNamara P, Curtis AM, Boston RC, Panda S, Hogenesch JB, Fitzgerald GA. BMAL1 and CLOCK, two essential components of the circadian clock, are involved in glucose homeostasis. *PloS Biol.* 2004 Nov;2(11):e377. doi: 10.1371/journal.pbio.0020377. Epub 2004 Nov 2.

15. Panda S, Antoch MP, Miller BH, Su AI, Schook AB, Straume M, Schultz PG, Kay SA, Takahashi JS, Hogenesch JB. Coordinated transcription of key pathways in the mouse by the circadian clock. *Cell.* 2002 May 3;109(3):307–20. doi: 10.1016/s0092-8674(02)00722-5.

16. Acosta-Rodriguez VA et al. Mice under caloric restriction self-impose a temporal restriction of food intake as revealed by an automated feeder system. *Cell Metab.* 2017;26(1):267–77.e2.

17. Chaix A, Lin T, Le HD, Chang MW, Panda S. Time-Restricted Feeding Prevents

Obesity and Metabolic Syndrome in Mice Lacking a Circadian Clock. *Cell Metab.* 2019 Feb 5;29(2):303–319.e4. doi: 10.1016/j.cmet.2018.08.004. Epub 2018 Aug 30.

18. Gill S, Panda S. A smartphone app reveals erratic diurnal eating patterns in humans that can be modulated for health benefits. *Cell Metab.* 2015;22(5):789–98.

19. Garaulet M et al. Timing of food intake predicts weight loss effectiveness. *Int J Obes.* 2013;37(4):604–11.

20. Sutton EF, Beyl R, Early KS, Cefalu WT, Ravussin E, Peterson CM. Early Time-Restricted Feeding Improves Insulin Sensitivity, Blood Pressure, and Oxidative Stress Even without Weight Loss in Men with Prediabetes. *Cell Metab.* 2018 Jun 5;27(6):1212–1221.e3. doi: 10.1016/j.cmet.2018.04.010. Epub 2018 May 10.

21. Wilkinson MJ, Manoogian ENC, Zadourian A, Lo H, Fakhouri S, Shoghi A, Wang X, Fleischer JG, Navlakha S, Panda S, Taub PR. Ten-Hour Time-Restricted Eating Reduces Weight, Blood Pressure, and Atherogenic Lipids in Patients with Metabolic Syndrome. *Cell Metab.* 2020 Jan 7;31(1):92–104.e5. doi: 10.1016/j.cmet.2019.11.004. Epub 2019 Dec 5.

22. Zomer E, Gurusamy K, Leach R, Trimmer C, Lobstein T, Morris S, James WPT, Finer N. Interventions that cause weight loss and the impact on cardiovascular risk factors: a systematic review and meta-analysis. *Obesity Rev.* 2016;17(10):1001–11.

23. Watanabe M et al. Bile acids induce energy expenditure by promoting intracellular thyroid hormone activation. *Nature* 2006;439(7075):484–89.

24. Chaix A et al. Time-restricted feeding is a preventative and therapeutic intervention against diverse nutritional challenges. *Cell Metab.* 2014;20(6):991–1005.

25. Hopkins PN. Molecular biology of atherosclerosis. *Physiol Rev.* 2013;93(3):1317–542.

## CHAPTER 4

1. Mohren DC et al. Prevalence of common infections among employees in different work schedules. *J Occupat Environ Med.* 2002;44(11):1003–11.

2. Greer S, Goldstein A., Walker M. The impact of sleep deprivation on food desire in the human brain. *Nat Commun.* 2013;4(2259). https://doi.org/10.1038/ncomms3259.

3. Chalernvanichakorn T, Sithisarankul P, Hiransuthikul N. Shift work and type 2 diabetic patients' health. *J Med Assoc Thai.* 2008 Jul;91(7):1093–96.

4. Chetty R, Stepner M, Abraham S, et al. The association between income and life expectancy in the United States, 2001–2014. *JAMA* 2016;315(16):1750–66. doi:10.1001/jama.2016.4226.

5. Althoff T, Sosič R, Hicks J, et al. Large-scale physical activity data reveal worldwide activity inequality. *Nature* 2017;547:336–39. https://doi.org/10.1038/nature23018.

6. Dunster GP, de la Iglesia L, Ben-Hamo M, Nave C, Fleischer JG, Panda S, de la Iglesia HO. Sleep more in Seattle: later school start times are associated with more sleep and better performance in high school students. *Sci. Adv.* 2018 Dec 12;4(12):eaau6200. doi: 10.1126/sciadv.aau6200.

7. Kellar D, Craft S. Brain insulin resistance in Alzheimer's disease and related disorders:

mechanisms and therapeutic approaches. *Lancet Neurol.* 2020 Sep;19(9):758–66. doi: 10.1016/S1474-4422(20)30231-3. Epub 2020 Jul 27.

8. Van Cauter E, Polonsky KS, Scheen AJ. Roles of circadian rhythmicity and sleep in human glucose regulation. *Endocrinol Rev.* 1997 Oct;18(5):716–38. doi: 10.1210/edrv.18.5.0317.

9. Gill S, Panda S. A smartphone app reveals erratic diurnal eating patterns in humans that can be modulated for health benefits. *Cell Metab.* 2015;22(5):789–98.

10. Gupta NJ, Kumar V, Panda S. A camera-phone based study reveals erratic eating pattern and disrupted daily eating-fasting cycle among adults in India. *PLoS ONE.* 2017;12(3):e0172852.

11. Ohayon M et al. National Sleep Foundation's sleep quality recommendations: first report. *Sleep Health.* 2017;3(1):6–19.

12. Hirshkowitz M et al. National Sleep Foundation's sleep time duration recommendations: methodology and results summary. *Sleep Health.* 2015;1(1):40–43.

13. Hirshkowitz M et al. National Sleep Foundation's updated sleep duration recommendations: final report. *Sleep Health.* 2015;1(4):233–43.

14. Dixon JB, O'Brien PEe. Health outcomes of severely obese type 2 diabetic subjects 1 year after laparoscopic adjustable gastric banding. *Diabetes Care.* 2002 Feb;25(2):358–63. doi: 10.2337/diacare.25.2.358.

## CHAPTER 5

1. Diabetes Prevention Program (DPP) Research Group. The Diabetes Prevention Program (DPP): description of lifestyle intervention. *Diabetes Care.* 2002 Dec;25(12):2165–71. doi: 10.2337/diacare.25.12.2165.

2. Carter S, Clifton PM, Keogh JB. Effect of intermittent compared with continuous energy restricted diet on glycemic control in patients with type 2 diabetes: a randomized noninferiority trial. *JAMA Netw Open.* 2018 Jul 6;1(3):e180756. doi: 10.1001/jamanetworkopen.2018.0756.

3. Cienfuegos S, Gabel K, Kalam F, Ezpeleta M, Wiseman E, Pavlou V, Lin S, Oliveira ML, Varady KA. Effects of 4- and 6-h time-restricted feeding on weight and cardiometabolic health: a randomized controlled trial in adults with obesity. *Cell Metab.* 2020 Sep 1;32(3):366–378.e3. doi: 10.1016/j.cmet.2020.06.018. Epub 2020 Jul 15.

4. Chow LS, Manoogian ENC, Alvear A, Fleischer JG, Thor H, Dietsche K, Wang Q, Hodges JS, Esch N, Malaeb S, Harindhanavudhi T, Nair KS, Panda S, Mashek DG. Time-restricted eating effects on body composition and metabolic measures in humans who are overweight: a feasibility study. *Obesity* (Silver Spring). 2020 May;28(5):860–69. doi: 10.1002/oby.22756. Epub 2020 Apr 9.

5. Carter S, Clifton PM, Keogh JB. Effect of intermittent compared with continuous energy restricted diet on glycemic control in patients with type 2 diabetes: a randomized noninferiority trial. *JAMA Netw Open.* 2018 Jul 6;1(3):e180756. doi: 10.1001/jamanetworkopen.2018.0756.

6. Kant AK, Graubard BI. 40-year trends in meal and snack eating behaviors of American adults. *J Acad Nutr Dietetics.* 2015;115(1):50–63.

7. Gill S, Panda S. A smartphone app reveals erratic diurnal eating patterns in humans that can be modulated for health benefits. *Cell Metab.* 2015;22(5):789–98.

8. Gupta NJ, Kumar V, Panda S. A camera-phone based study reveals erratic eating pattern and disrupted daily eating-fasting cycle among adults in India. *PLoS ONE.* 2017;12(3):e0172852.

9. Jakubowicz D, Landau Z, Tsameret S, Wainstein J, Raz I, Ahren B, Chapnik N, Barnea M, Ganz T, Menaged M, Mor N, Bar-Dayan Y, Froy O. Reduction in glycated hemoglobin and daily insulin dose alongside circadian clock upregulation in patients with type 2 diabetes consuming a three-meal diet: a randomized clinical trial. *Diabetes Care.* 2019 Dec;42(12):2171–80. doi: 10.2337/dc19-1142. Epub 2019 Sep 23.

10. Kahleova H, Belinova L, Malinska H, et al. Eating two larger meals a day (breakfast and lunch) is more effective than six smaller meals in a reduced-energy regimen for patients with type 2 diabetes: a randomised crossover study. *Diabetologia* 2014;57:1552–60. https://doi.org/10.1007/s00125-014-3253-5.

11. Garaulet M, Gómez-Abellán P, Alburquerque-Béjar JJ, Lee YC, Ordovás JM, Scheer FA. Timing of food intake predicts weight loss effectiveness. *Int J Obes* (London). 2013 Apr;37(4):604–11. doi: 10.1038/ijo.2012.229. Epub 2013 Jan 29. Erratum in: *Int J Obes* (London). 2013 Apr;37(4):624.

12. Stunkard AJ, Grace WJ, Wolff HG. The night-eating syndrome; a pattern of food intake among certain obese patients. *Am J Med.* 1955 Jul;19(1):78–86. doi: 10.1016/0002-9343(55)90276-x.

13. Takeda E, Terao J, Nakaya Y, Miyamoto K, Baba Y, Chuman H, Kaji R, Ohmori T, Rokutan K. Stress control and human nutrition. *J Med Invest.* 2004 Aug;51(3-4):139–45. doi: 10.2152/jmi.51.139.

14. Liu Z et al. PER1 phosphorylation specifies feeding rhythm in mice. *Cell Rep.* 2014;7(5):1509–20.

## CHAPTER 6

1. Yancy WS Jr, Foy M, Chalecki AM, Vernon MC, Westman EC. A low-carbohydrate, ketogenic diet to treat type 2 diabetes. *Nutr Metab* (London). 2005 Dec 1;2:34. doi: 10.1186/1743-7075-2-34.

2. Chaix A, Zarrinpar A, Miu P, Panda S. Time-restricted feeding is a preventative and therapeutic intervention against diverse nutritional challenges. *Cell Metab.* 2014 Dec 2;20(6):991–1005. doi: 10.1016/j.cmet.2014.11.001.

3. Crosby P, Hamnett R, Putker M, Hoyle NP, Reed M, Karam CJ, Maywood ES, Stangherlin A, Chesham JE, Hayter EA, Rosenbrier-Ribeiro L, Newham P, Clevers H, Bechtold DA, O'Neill JS. Insulin/IGF-1 drives PERIOD synthesis to entrain circadian rhythms with feeding time. *Cell.* 2019 May 2;177(4):896–909.e20. doi: 10.1016/j.cell.2019.02.017. Epub 2019 Apr 25.

4. https://www.wsj.com/graphics/what-americans-should-eat-dietary-guidelines.

5. Suez J, Korem T, Zeevi D, Zilberman-Schapira G, Thaiss CA, Maza O, Israeli D, Zmora N, Gilad S, Weinberger A, Kuperman Y, Harmelin A, Kolodkin-Gal I, Shapiro H, Halpern Z, Segal E, Elinav E. Artificial sweeteners induce glucose intol-

erance by altering the gut microbiota. *Nature.* 2014 Oct 9;514(7521):181–86. doi: 10.1038/nature13793. Epub 2014 Sep 17.

6. Estruch R, Martínez-González MA, Corella D, Salas-Salvadó J, Ruiz-Gutiérrez V, Covas MI, Fiol M, Gómez-Gracia E, López-Sabater MC, Vinyoles E, Arós F, Conde M, Lahoz C, Lapetra J, Sáez G, Ros E; PREDIMED Study Investigators. Effects of a Mediterranean-style diet on cardiovascular risk factors: a randomized trial. *Ann Intern Med.* 2006 Jul 4;145(1):1–11. doi: 10.7326/0003-4819-145-1-2006 07040-00004. Erratum in: *Ann Intern Med.* 2018 Aug 21;169(4):270–271.

7. Castro-Diehl C, Wood AC, Redline S, Reid M, Johnson DA, Maras JE, Jacobs DR Jr, Shea S, Crawford A, St-Onge MP. Mediterranean diet pattern and sleep duration and insomnia symptoms in the Multi-Ethnic Study of Atherosclerosis. *Sleep.* 2018 Nov 1;41(11):zsy158. doi: 10.1093/sleep/zsy158.

8. Hall KD, Ayuketah A, Brychta R, Cai H, Cassimatis T, Chen KY, Chung ST, Costa E, Courville A, Darcey V, Fletcher LA, Forde CG, Gharib AM, Guo J, Howard R, Joseph PV, McGehee S, Ouwerkerk R, Raisinger K, Rozga I, Stagliano M, Walter M, Walter PJ, Yang S, Zhou M. Ultra-processed diets cause excess calorie intake and weight gain: an inpatient randomized controlled trial of ad libitum food intake. *Cell Metab.* 2020 Oct 6;32(4):690. doi: 10.1016/j.cmet.2020.08.014. Erratum for: *Cell Metab.* 2019 Jul 2;30(1):67–77.e3.

9. Jakubowicz D, Wainstein J, Landau Z, Ahren B, Barnea M, Bar-Dayan Y, Froy O. High-energy breakfast based on whey protein reduces body weight, postprandial glycemia and HbA1c in type 2 diabetes. *J Nutr Biochem.* 2017 Nov;49:1–7. doi: 10.1016/j.jnutbio.2017.07.005. Epub 2017 Jul 21.

10. https://www.wsj.com/graphics/what-americans-should-eat-dietary-guidelines.

11. Deer RR, Volpi E. Protein intake and muscle function in older adults. *Curr Opin Clin Nutr Metab Care.* 2015 May;18(3):248–53. doi: 10.1097/MCO.0000000000000162.

## CHAPTER 7

1. De Cabo R, Mattson MP. Effects of intermittent fasting on health, aging, and disease. *N Engl J Med.* 2019 Dec 26;381(26):2541–51. doi: 10.1056/NEJMra1905136. Erratum in: *N Engl J Med.* 2020 Jan 16;382(3):298. Erratum in: *N Engl J Med.* 2020 Mar 5;382(10):978.

2. Schellenberg ES, Dryden DM, Vandermeer B, Ha C, Korownyk C. Lifestyle interventions for patients with and at risk for type 2 diabetes: a systematic review and meta-analysis. *Ann Intern Med.* 2013;159:543–51.

3. Chen L, Pei JH, Kuang J, et al. Effect of lifestyle intervention in patients with type 2 diabetes: a meta-analysis. *Metabolism.* 2015;64:338–47.

4. Lin X, Zhang X, Guo J, et al. Effects of exercise training on cardiorespiratory fitness and biomarkers of cardiometabolic health: a systematic review and meta-analysis of randomized controlled trials. *J Am Heart Assoc.* 2015;4:4.

5. Yardley JE, Hay J, Abou-Setta AM, Marks SD, McGavock J. A systematic review and meta-analysis of exercise interventions in adults with type 1 diabetes. *Diabetes Res Clin Pract.* 2014;106:393–400.

6. Sylow L, Kleinert M, Richter EA, Jensen TE. Exercise-stimulated glucose uptake—regulation and implications for glycaemic control. *Nat Rev Endocrinol.* 2017 Mar;13(3):133–48. doi: 10.1038/nrendo.2016.162. Epub 2016 Oct 14.

7. Snedeker JG, Gautieri A. The role of collagen crosslinks in ageing and diabetes—the good, the bad, and the ugly. *Muscles Ligaments Tendons J.* 2014 Nov 17;4(3):303–08.

8. Edgar DM et al. Influence of running wheel activity on free-running sleep/wake and drinking circadian rhythms in mice. *Physiol Behav.* 1991;50(2):373–78.

9. Brand S et al. High exercise levels are related to favorable sleep patterns and psychological functioning in adolescents: a comparison of athletes and controls. *J Adoles Heal.* 2010;46(2):133–41.

10. Reid KJ et al. Aerobic exercise improves self-reported sleep and quality of life in older adults with insomnia. *Sleep Med.* 2010;11(9):934–40.

11. Tworoger SS et al. Effects of a yearlong moderate-intensity exercise and a stretching intervention on sleep quality in postmenopausal women. *Sleep.* 2003;26(7):830–36.

12. Van Someren EJ et al. Long-term fitness training improves the circadian rest-activity rhythm in healthy elderly males. *J Biol Rhythms.* 1997;12(2):146–56.

13. Kubota T et al. Interleukin-15 and interleukin-2 enhance non-REM sleep in rabbits. *Am J Physiol:Regul Integ Comp Physiol.* 2001;281(3):R1004–12.

14. Li Y et al. Association of serum irisin concentrations with the presence and severity of obstructive sleep apnea syndrome. *J Clin Lab Anal.* 2016;31(5):e22077.

15. Awad KM et al. Exercise is associated with a reduced incidence of sleep-disordered breathing. *Am J Med.* 2012;125(5):485–90.

16. Sleiman SF, Henry J, Al-Haddad R, El Hayek L, Abou Haidar E, Stringer T, Ulja D, Karuppagounder SS, Holson EB, Ratan RR, Ninan I, Chao MV. Exercise promotes the expression of brain derived neurotrophic factor (BDNF) through the action of the ketone body β-hydroxybutyrate. *Elife.* 2016 Jun 2;5:e15092. doi: 10.7554/eLife .15092.

17. Atkinson G, Davenne D. Relationships between sleep, physical activity and human health. *Physiol Behav.* 2007 Feb 28;90(2-3):229–35. doi: 10.1016/j.physbeh.2006.09 .015. Epub 2006 Oct 25.

18. Yang N, Meng QJ. Circadian clocks in articular cartilage and bone: a compass in the sea of matrices. *J Biol Rhythms.* 2016;31(5):415–27.

19. Schroder EA et al. Intrinsic muscle clock is necessary for musculoskeletal health. *J Physiol.* 2015;593(24):5387–404.

20. Aoyama S, Shibata S. The role of circadian rhythms in muscular and osseous physiology and their regulation by nutrition and exercise. *Frontiers in Neurosci.* 2017;11: no. 63.

21. Woldt E et al. Rev-erb-α modulates skeletal muscle oxidative capacity by regulating mitochondrial biogenesis and autophagy. *Nature Med.* 2013;19(8):1039–46.

22. Thun E, Bjorvatn B, Flo E, Harris A, Pallesen S. Sleep, circadian rhythms, and athletic performance. *Sleep Med. Rev.* 2015 Oct;23:1–9. doi: 10.1016/j.smrv.2014.11.003. Epub 2014 Nov 20.

23. Chang J, Garva R, Pickard A, Yeung CC, Mallikarjun V, Swift J, Holmes DF, Calverley B, Lu Y, Adamson A, Raymond-Hayling H, Jensen O, Shearer T, Meng

QJ, Kadler KE. Circadian control of the secretory pathway maintains collagen homeostasis. *Nat Cell Biol.* 2020 Jan;22(1):74–86. doi: 10.1038/s41556-019-0441-z. Epub 2020 Jan 6.

24. Steidle-Kloc E et al. Does exercise training impact clock genes in patients with coronary artery disease and type 2 diabetes mellitus? *Eur J Prev Card.* 2016;23(13): 1375–82.

25. Chimen M, Kennedy A, Nirantharakumar K, Pang TT, Andrews R, Narendran P. What are the health benefits of physical activity in type 1 diabetes mellitus? A literature review. *Diabetologia.* 2012;55:542–51.

26. Snowling NJ, Hopkins WG. Effects of different modes of exercise training on glucose control and risk factors for complications in type 2 diabetic patients: a meta-analysis. *Diabetes Care* 2006;29:2518–27.

27. Jelleyman C, Yates T, O'Donovan G, et al. The effects of high-intensity interval training on glucose regulation and insulin resistance: a meta-analysis. *Obes Rev.* 2015;16:942–61.

28. Tonoli C, Heyman E, Roelands B, et al. Effects of different types of acute and chronic (training) exercise on glycaemic control in type 1 diabetes mellitus: a meta-analysis. *Sports Med.* 2012;42:1059–80.

29. Innes KE, Selfe TK. Yoga for adults with type 2 diabetes: a systematic review of controlled trials. *J Diabetes Res.* 2016;2016:6979370.

30. Ahn S, Song R. Effects of tai chi exercise on glucose control, neuropathy scores, balance, and quality of life in patients with type 2 diabetes and neuropathy. *J Alt Complement Med.* 2012;18:1172–78.

31. Althoff T et al. Large-scale physical activity data reveal worldwide activity inequality. *Nature* 2017;547(7663):336–39.

32. Bassett DR, Schneider PL, Huntington GE. Physical activity in an Old Order Amish community. *Med Sci Sports and Exercise.* 2004;36(1):79–85.

33. De la Iglesia HO et al. Access to electric light is associated with shorter sleep duration in a traditionally hunter-gatherer community. *J Biol Rhythms.* 2015; 30(4):342–50.

34. Van Praag H et al. Running enhances neurogenesis, learning, and long-term potentiation in mice. *Proc Nat Acad Sci USA.* 1999;96(23):13427–31.

35. Van Marken Lichtenbelt WD et al. Cold-activated brown adipose tissue in healthy men. *N Eng J Med.* 2009;360(15):1500–08.

36. Ouellet V, et al. Brown adipose tissue oxidative metabolism contributes to energy expenditure during acute cold exposure in humans. *J Clin Invest.* 2012;122(2):545–52.

37. Pasieka AM, Rafacho A. Impact of glucocorticoid excess on glucose tolerance: clinical and preclinical evidence. *Metabolites.* 2016 Aug 3;6(3):24. doi: 10.3390/metabo 6030024.

38. Thun E et al. Sleep, circadian rhythms, and athletic performance. *Sleep Med Rev.* 2015;23: 1–9.

39. King NA, Burley VJ, Blundell JE. Exercise-induced suppression of appetite: effects on food intake and implications for energy balance. *Eur J Clin Nutr.* 1994;48(10): 715–24.

40. Richter EA, Hargreaves M. Exercise, GLUT4, and skeletal muscle glucose uptake. *Phys Rev.* 2013;93(3):993–1017.

41. Van Cauter E et al. Nocturnal decrease in glucose tolerance during constant glucose infusion. *J Clin Endocrin Metab.* 1989;69(3):604–11.

42. Sturis J et al. 24-hour glucose profiles during continuous or oscillatory insulin infusion: demonstration of the functional significance of ultradian insulin oscillations. *J Clin Invest.* 1995;95(4):1464–71.

43. Chaix A et al. Time-restricted feeding is a preventative and therapeutic intervention against diverse nutritional challenges. *Cell Metab.* 2014;20(6):991–1005.

44. King NA, Burley VJ, Blundell JE. Exercise-induced suppression of appetite: effects on food intake and implications for energy balance. *Eur J Clin Nutr.* 1994 Oct;48(10):715–24.

## CHAPTER 8

1. Grandner MA, Seixas A, Shetty S, Shenoy S. Sleep duration and diabetes risk: population trends and potential mechanisms. *Curr Diab Rep.* 2016 Nov;16(11):106. doi: 10.1007/s11892-016-0805-8.

2. Spiegel K, Leproult R, Van Cauter E. Impact of sleep debt on metabolic and endocrine function. *Lancet.* 1999 Oct 23;354(9188):1435–39. doi: 10.1016/S0140-6736(99)01376-8.

3. Wu JC, Gillin JC, Buchsbaum MS, Hershey T, Hazlett E, Sicotte N, Bunney WE Jr. The effect of sleep deprivation on cerebral glucose metabolic rate in normal humans assessed with positron emission tomography. *Sleep.* 1991 Apr;14(2):155–62.

4. De Havas JA, Parimal S, Soon CS, Chee MW. Sleep deprivation reduces default mode network connectivity and anti-correlation during rest and task performance. *Neuroimage.* 2012 Jan 16;59(2):1745–51. doi: 10.1016/j.neuroimage.2011.08.026. Epub 2011 Aug 18.

5. Gujar N, Yoo SS, Hu P, Walker MP. The unrested resting brain: sleep deprivation alters activity within the default-mode network. *J Cogn Neurosci.* 2010 Aug;22(8):1637–48. doi: 10.1162/jocn.2009.21331.

6. Xie L, Kang H, Xu Q, Chen MJ, Liao Y, Thiyagarajan M, O'Donnell J, Christensen DJ, Nicholson C, Iliff JJ, Takano T, Deane R, Nedergaard M. Sleep drives metabolite clearance from the adult brain. *Science.* 2013 Oct 18;342(6156):373–77. doi: 10.1126/science.1241224.

7. Mestre H, Mori Y, Nedergaard M. The brain's glymphatic system: current controversies. *Trends Neurosci.* 2020 Jul;43(7):458–66. doi: 10.1016/j.tins.2020.04.003. Epub 2020 May 15.

8. Benedict C, Brooks SJ, O'Daly OG, Almèn MS, Morell A, Åberg K, Gingnell M, Schultes B, Hallschmid M, Broman JE, Larsson EM, Schiöth HB. Acute sleep deprivation enhances the brain's response to hedonic food stimuli: an fMRI study. *J Clin Endocrinol Metab.* 2012 Mar;97(3):E443–7. doi: 10.1210/jc.2011-2759. Epub 2012 Jan 18.

9. Redwine L, Hauger RL, Gillin JC, Irwin M. Effects of sleep and sleep deprivation on interleukin-6, growth hormone, cortisol, and melatonin levels in humans. J Clin Endocrinol Metab. 2000 Oct;85(10):3597–603. doi: 10.1210/jcem.85.10.6871.

10. McHill AW et al. Impact of circadian misalignment on energy metabolism during simulated nightshift work. Proc Nat Acad Sci USA. 2014;111(48):17302–07.

11. Grandner MA, Seixas A, Shetty S, Shenoy S. Sleep duration and diabetes risk: population trends and potential mechanisms. Curr Diab Rep. 2016 Nov;16(11):106. doi: 10.1007/s11892-016-0805-8.

12. Leproult R, Copinschi G, Buxton O, Van Cauter E. Sleep loss results in an elevation of cortisol levels the next evening. Sleep. 1997 Oct;20(10):865–70.

13. McAlpine CS, Kiss MG, Rattik S, He S, Vassalli A, Valet C, Anzai A, Chan CT, Mindur JE, Kahles F, Poller WC, Frodermann V, Fenn AM, Gregory AF, Halle L, Iwamoto Y, Hoyer FF, Binder CJ, Libby P, Tafti M, Scammell TE, Nahrendorf M, Swirski FK. Sleep modulates haematopoiesis and protects against atherosclerosis. Nature. 2019 Feb;566(7744):383–87. doi: 10.1038/s41586-019-0948-2. Epub 2019 Feb 13.

14. Irwin MR, Olmstead R, Carroll JE. Sleep disturbance, sleep duration, and inflammation: a systematic review and meta-analysis of cohort studies and experimental sleep deprivation. Biol Psychiatry. 2016 Jul 1;80(1):40–52. doi: 10.1016/j.biopsych.2015.05.014. Epub 2015 Jun 1.

15. Gaspar LS et al. Obstructive sleep apnea and hallmarks of aging. Trends Mol Med. 2017;23(8):675–92.

16. Reichmuth KJ, Austin D, Skatrud JB, Young T. Association of sleep apnea and type II diabetes: a population-based study. Am J Respir Crit Care Med. 2005 Dec 15;172(12):1590–95. doi: 10.1164/rccm.200504-637OC. Epub 2005 Sep 28.

17. Dawson A, Abel SL, Loving RT, Dailey G, Shadan FF, Cronin JW, Kripke DF, Kline LE. CPAP therapy of obstructive sleep apnea in type 2 diabetics improves glycemic control during sleep. J Clin Sleep Med. 2008 Dec 15;4(6):538–42.

18. Kronfeld-Schor N, Einat H. Circadian rhythms and depression: human psychopathology and animal models. Neuropharm. 2012;62(1):101–14.

19. Coles ME, Schubert JR, Nota JA. Sleep, circadian rhythms, and anxious traits. Curr Psych Rep. 2015;17(9):73.

20. Kripke DF et al. Mortality associated with sleep duration and insomnia. Arch Gen Psych. 2002;59(2):131–36.

21. Hirshkowitz M et al. National Sleep Foundation's sleep time duration recommendations: methodology and results summary. Sleep Health. 2015;1(1):40–43.

22. Hirshkowitz M et al. National Sleep Foundation's updated sleep duration recommendations: final report. Sleep Health. 2015;1(4):233–43.

23. Hansen AL, Dahl L, Olson G, Thornton D, Graff IE, Frøyland L, Thayer JF, Pallesen S. Fish consumption, sleep, daily functioning, and heart rate variability. J Clin Sleep Med. 2014 May 15;10(5):567–75. doi: 10.5664/jcsm.3714.

24. Rondanelli M, Opizzi A, Monteferrario F, Antoniello N, Manni R, Klersy C. The effect of melatonin, magnesium, and zinc on primary insomnia in long-term care fa-

cility residents in Italy: a double-blind, placebo-controlled clinical trial. *J Am Geriatr Soc.* 2011 Jan;59(1):82–90. doi: 10.1111/j.1532-5415.2010.03232.x.

25. Muscogiuri G, Barrea L, Aprano S, Framondi L, Di Matteo R, Laudisio D, Pugliese G, Savastano S, Colao A, on behalf of the Opera Prevention Project. Sleep quality in obesity: does adherence to the Mediterranean diet matter? *Nutrients.* 2020 May 10;12(5):1364. doi: 10.3390/nu12051364.

26. Gill S, Panda S. A smartphone app reveals erratic diurnal eating patterns in humans that can be modulated for health benefits. *Cell Metab.* 2015;22(5):789–98.

27. Wilkinson MJ, Manoogian ENC, Zadourian A, Lo H, Fakhouri S, Shoghi A, Wang X, Fleischer JG, Navlakha S, Panda S, Taub PR. Ten-hour time-restricted eating reduces weight, blood pressure, and atherogenic lipids in patients with metabolic syndrome. *Cell Metab.* 2020 Jan 7;31(1):92–104.e5. doi: 10.1016/j.cmet.2019.11.004. Epub 2019 Dec 5.

28. Martin B, Mattson MP, Maudsley S. Caloric restriction and intermittent fasting: two potential diets for successful brain aging. *Ageing Res Rev.* 2006;5( 3):332–53.

29. Hatori M, Panda S. The emerging roles of melanopsin in behavioral adaptation to light. *Trends Mol Med.* 2010 Oct;16(10):435–46. doi: 10.1016/j.molmed.2010.07.005. Epub 2010 Aug 31.

30. Takasu NN, Hashimoto S, Yamanaka Y, Tanahashi Y, Yamazaki A, Honma S, Honma K. Repeated exposures to daytime bright light increase nocturnal melatonin rise and maintain circadian phase in young subjects under fixed sleep schedule. *Am J Physiol Regul Integr Comp Physiol.* 2006 Dec;291(6):R1799–807. doi: 10.1152/ajpregu.00211.2006. Epub 2006 Jul 13.

31. Viola AU, James LM, Schlangen LJ, Dijk DJ. Blue-enriched white light in the workplace improves self-reported alertness, performance and sleep quality. *Scand J Work Environ Health.* 2008 Aug;34(4):297–306. doi: 10.5271/sjweh.1268. Epub 2008 Sep 22.

32. Burkhart K, Phelps JR. Amber lenses to block blue light and improve sleep: a randomized trial. *Chronobiol Int.* 2009 Dec;26(8):1602–12. doi: 10.3109/07420520903 523719.

33. Ferracioli-Oda E, Qawasmi A, Bloch MH. Meta-analysis: melatonin for the treatment of primary sleep disorders. *PLoS ONE.* 2013;8(5):e63773.

34. Lin CL, Yeh MC, Harnod T, Lin CL, Kao CH. Risk of Type 2 diabetes in patients with nonapnea sleep disorders in using different types of hypnotics: a population-based retrospective cohort study. *Medicine* (Baltimore). 2015 Sep;94(38):e1621. doi: 10.1097/MD.0000000000001621.

## CHAPTER 9

1. Lim S, Bae JH, Kwon HS, Nauck MA. COVID-19 and diabetes mellitus: from pathophysiology to clinical management. *Nat Rev Endocrinol.* 2021 Jan;17(1):11–30. doi: 10.1038/s41574-020-00435-4. Epub 2020 Nov 13.

2. Black JA, Simmons RK, Boothby CE, Davies MJ, Webb D, Khunti K, Long GH,

Griffin SJ. Medication burden in the first 5 years following diagnosis of type 2 diabetes: findings from the ADDITION-UK trial cohort. *BMJ Open Diabetes Res Care.* 2015 Oct 1;3(1):e000075. doi: 10.1136/bmjdrc-2014-000075.

3. Reinberg A, Lévi F. Clinical chronopharmacology with special reference to NSAIDs. *Scand J Rheumatol Suppl.* 1987;65:118–22. doi: 10.3109/03009748709102189.

4. Buttgereit F, Doering G, Schaeffler A, Witte S, Sierakowski S, Gromnica-Ihle E, Jeka S, Krueger K, Szechinski J, Alten R. Efficacy of modified-release versus standard prednisone to reduce duration of morning stiffness of the joints in rheumatoid arthritis (CAPRA-1): a double-blind, randomised controlled trial. *Lancet.* 2008 Jan 19;371(9608):205–14. doi: 10.1016/S0140-6736(08)60132-4.

5. Hermida RC, Crespo JJ, Domínguez-Sardiña M, Otero A, Moyá A, Ríos MT, Sineiro E, Castiñeira MC, Callejas PA, Pousa L, Salgado JL, Durán C, Sánchez JJ, Fernández JR, Mojón A, Ayala DE; Hygia Project Investigators. Bedtime hypertension treatment improves cardiovascular risk reduction: the Hygia Chronotherapy Trial. *Eur Heart J.* 2020 Dec 21;41(48):4565–76. doi: 10.1093/eurheartj/ehz754.

6. Wilkinson MJ, Manoogian ENC, Zadourian A, Lo H, Fakhouri S, Shoghi A, Wang X, Fleischer JG, Navlakha S, Panda S, Taub PR. Ten-hour time-restricted eating reduces weight, blood pressure, and atherogenic lipids in patients with metabolic syndrome. *Cell Metab.* 2020 Jan 7;31(1):92–104.e5. doi: 10.1016/j.cmet.2019.11.004. Epub 2019 Dec 5.

7. Hutchison AT, Regmi P, Manoogian ENC, Fleischer JG, Wittert GA, Panda S, Heilbronn LK. Time-restricted feeding improves glucose tolerance in men at risk for type 2 diabetes: a randomized crossover trial. *Obesity* (Silver Spring). 2019 May;27(5):724–32. doi: 10.1002/oby.22449. Epub 2019 Apr 19.

8. Poolsup N, Suksomboon N, Kyaw AM. Systematic review and meta-analysis of the effectiveness of continuous glucose monitoring (CGM) on glucose control in diabetes. *Diabetol Metab Syndr.* 2013 Jul 23;5:39. doi: 10.1186/1758-5996-5-39.

## CHAPTER 10

1. https://www.cdc.gov/healthyweight/assessing/index.html.

# INDEX

# ABOUT THE AUTHOR

**Satchin Panda, PhD,** is a leading expert in the field of circadian rhythm research. He is a professor at the Salk Institute for Biological Studies and a founding executive member of the Center for Circadian Biology at the University of California, San Diego. Dr. Panda is a Pew Biomedical Scholar and a recipient of the Julie Martin Mid-Career Award in Aging Research. As a recognition of the impact of his work regarding circadian rhythms and diabetes, Dr. Panda has been invited to speak at conferences around the world, including Diabetes UK, the American Diabetes Association, the Danish Diabetes Association, and the respective professional diabetes societies of Europe and Australia.